60+ Health Careers You Should Know About

A GUIDE TO HELP YOU START YOUR HEALTH CAREER

WRITTEN BY
DR AISHA HARRIS, MD

60+ Health Careers You Should Know About

Published by BLK FAM DOC
432 N Saginaw St, Suite 401A
Flint, MI 48502

ISBN: 979-8-9889390-0-9

Printed by IngramSpark, Inc., in the United States of America.

First printing, 2023.

www.blkfamdoc.com

This book is dedicated to the people who have a passion for helping others and the community of loved ones that support those dreams and ambitions.

ABOUT THE AUTHOR

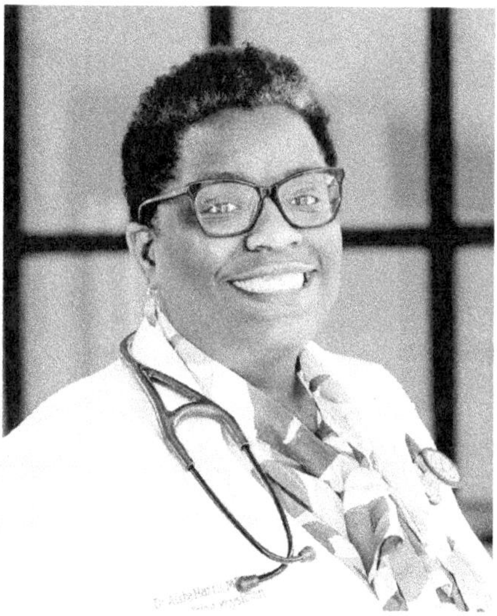

Dr Aisha Harris, MD is a board certified Family Medicine Physician who is the owner of Harris Family Health, a direct primary care clinic in her hometown of Flint, Michigan.

She earned a Bachelor's of Science in Chemical Engineering from the University of Michigan and graduated from Georgetown University School of Medicine with a Doctorate in Medicine. She trained at the University of Illinois in Chicago Family Medicine residency program.

Dr Harris is a Family Medicine Physician that focuses on improving health literacy and health access through outreach work. She also does public health and health advocacy work within various organizations to help address health disparities.

Dr Aisha Harris, MD

Family Medicine Physician
Harris Family Health

TABLE OF CONTENTS

Introduction

The purpose of this book is to expand the readers understanding of the diverse and different health careers they may potentially be interested in. Through this guide readers will be able to understand more about each health career and have a better foundation for their future decisions to pursue a career in healthcare.

This book is an introduction to many health careers and will help develop the framework to explore and learn more about specific health careers through other resources. Starting with this guide expands the reader's perspective and hopefully increases the number of health professionals and individuals in health related fields.

Too often people are not aware of the variety of career options in different areas, including healthcare, so "60+ Health Careers You Should Know About" is a great resource to start a career in health or shift into another career in health.

Review the various health career summaries and learn more about the clinical and non-clinical career options that are essential for our health system to provide quality care and improve quality of life.

ALPHABETICAL CAREER LIST

ALPHABETICAL CAREER LIST

60+ HEALTH CAREERS YOU SHOULD KNOW ABOUT

ALPHABETICAL CAREER LIST

DEFINITIONS

Overview: General overview of the occupation's general description and responsibilities.

Education Levels: Typical level of education that most workers need to enter the occupation.

- Associate's Degree: 2 years of school
- Bachelor's Degree: 4 years of school
- Master's Degree: 2+ years of school after a Bachelor's Degree
- Doctorate Degree: 3+ years of school after earning a Bachelor's or Master's degree
- Internship Training: 1 year of training after earning a degree
- Residency Training: 2+ years of training after earning a Doctorate degree
- Fellowship Training: 1+ years of subspecialized training after completing a Residency training

Type of Area:

- **Clinical:** An occupation that provides direct patient care.
- **Non-Clinical:** An occupation that does not provide direct patient care.

State License or Certification: Occupations that have indicated a state license or formal certification is needed in order to work in the occupation.

Average Salary and Hourly Range: The average salary and hourly for the occupation.

Salary Range: The range from the lowest 10 percent of people in the occupation to the highest 10 percent earned of people in the occupation.

Number of Jobs in 2021: The number of people employed in the occupation in 2021.

Job Outlook: The projected percent change in employment from 2021 to 2031. The average growth rate for all occupations is 5 percent.

10 Year Change 2021-2023: The projected numeric change in employment from 2021 to 2031.

Work Environment: The largest employers for the occupation.

CLINICAL CAREERS

Art Therapists
Athletic Trainers
Audiologists
Cardiovascular Technologists and Technicians
Chiropractors
Clinical Laboratory Technologists and Technicians
Community Health Workers
Diagnostic Medical Sonographers
Dental Assistants
Dental Hygienists
Dentists
Dietitian Nutritionists
Emergency Medical Technician and Paramedics
Estheticians and Skincare Specialists
Exercise Physiologists
Health Education Specialists
Health Information Technologists and Medical Registra
Home Health and Personal Care Aides
Licensed Practical and Licensed Vocational Nurses
Massage Therapists
Medical Assistants
MRI Technologists
Music Therapists
Nuclear Medicine Technologists
Nurse Anesthetists
Nurse Assistants
Nurse Midwives
Nurse Practitioners
Occupational Therapists
Occupational Therapy Assistants

CLINICAL CAREERS

Opticians
Optometrists
Orthotists and Prosthetists
Pharmacists
Pharmacy Technicians
Phlebotomists
Physical Therapists
Physical Therapist Assistants
Physician and Surgeons
Physician Assistants
Podiatrists
Psychiatric Technicians
Radiation Therapists
Radiologic Technologists
Registered Nurses
Rehabilitation Counselors
Respiratory Therapists
Social Workers
Speech Language Pathologists
Surgical Technologists
Veterinarians
Veterinary Assistants and Laboratory Animal Caretakers
Veterinary Technologists and Technicians

NON-CLINICAL CAREERS

Biochemists and Biophysicists
Biological Technicians
Biomedical Engineers
Dental and Ophthalmic Laboratory Technicians and Medical Appliance Technicians
Epidemiologists
Health Information Technologists and Medical Registrar
Medical and Health Services Managers
Medical Records Specialists
Medical Scientists
Medical Transcriptionists
Wholesale and Manufacturing Sales Representatives

US NEWS BEST HEALTH CAREER JOBS 2023

1. **Nurse Practitioner**
2. **Physician Assistant**
3. **Physical Therapist**
4. **Dentist**
5. **Veterinarian**
6. **Physician**
7. **Orthodontist**
8. **Registered Nurse**
9. **Oral and Maxillofacial Surgeon (Physician)**
10. **Nurse Anesthetist**
11. **Speech Language Pathologist**
12. **Psychiatrist (Physician)**
13. **Optometrist**
14. **Pediatrician (Physician)**
15. **Respiratory Therapist**
16. **Anesthesiologist**
17. **Obstetrician and Gynecologist**
18. **Chiropractor**
19. **Prosthodontist**
20. **Occupational Therapist**
21. **Dietitian and Nutritionist**
22. **Pharmacist**
23. **Audiologist**
24. **Nurse Midwife**
25. **Esthetician and Skincare Specialist**

CAREERS BY EDUCATION LEVEL

High School Diploma

- **Community Health Workers**
- **Dental and Ophthalmic Laboratory Technicians and Medical Appliance Technicians**
- **Home Health and Personal Care Aides**
- **Opticians**
- **Pharmacy Technicians**
- **Veterinary Assistants and Laboratory Animal Caretakers**

Associate's Degree

- **Cardiovascular Technologists and Technicians**
- **Dental Hygienists**
- **Diagnostic Medical Sonographers**
- **Health Information Technologists and Medical Registrars**
- **MRI Technologists**
- **Nuclear Medicine Technologists**
- **Occupational Therapy Assistants**
- **Physical Therapist Assistants**
- **Radiation Therapists**
- **Radiologic Technologists**
- **Respiratory Therapists**
- **Veterinary Technologists and Technicians**

Postsecondary Non-Degree

- **Dental Assistants**
- **Emergency Medical Technician and Paramedics**
- **Esthetician and Skincare Specialists**
- **Licensed Practical and Licensed Vocational Nurses**
- **Massage Therapists**
- **Medical Assistants**
- **Medical Records Specialists**
- **Medical Transcriptionists**
- **Nursing Assistants**
- **Phlebotomists**
- **Psychiatric Technicians**
- **Surgical Technologists**

CAREERS BY EDUCATION LEVEL

Bachelor's Degree

- **Biological Technicians**
- **Biomedical Engineers**
- **Clinical Laboratory Technologists and Technicians**
- **Dietitian Nutritionists**
- **Exercise Physiologists**
- **Health Education Specialists**
- **Medical and Health Services Managers**
- **Music Therapists**
- **Registered Nurses**
- **Social Workers**
- **Wholesale and Manufacturing Sales Representatives**

Master's Degree

- **Art Therapists**
- **Athletic Trainers**
- **Epidemiologists**
- **Nurse Anesthetists**
- **Nurse Midwives**
- **Nurse Practitioners**
- **Occupational Therapists**
- **Orthotists and Prosthetists**
- **Physician Assistants**
- **Rehabilitation Counselors**
- **Speech Language Pathologists**

Doctorate Degree

- **Biochemists and Biophysicists**
- **Chiropractors**
- **Dentists**
- **Medical Scientists**
- **Optometrists**
- **Pharmacists**
- **Physical Therapists**
- **Physicians and Surgeons**
- **Podiatrists**
- **Veterinarians**

CAREERS BY JOB OUTOOK

Much Faster Than Average Growth (16-40%)

- **Athletic Trainers**
- **Biochemists and Biophysicists**
- **Epidemiologists**
- **Esthetician and Skincare Specialists**
- **Health Information Technologists and Medical Registrars**
- **Home Health and Personal Care Aides**
- **Massage Therapists**
- **Medical and Health Services Managers**
- **Medical Assistants**
- **Medical Scientists**
- **Nurse Anesthetists**
- **Nurse Midwives**
- **Nurse Practitioners**
- **Occupational Therapy Assistants**
- **Orthotists and Prosthetists**
- **Physical Therapists**
- **Physician Assistants**
- **Physical Therapist Assistants**
- **Respiratory Therapists**
- **Speech Language Pathologists**
- **Veterinarians**
- **Veterinary Assistants and Laboratory Animal Caretakers**
- **Veterinary Technologists and Technicians**

Job Outlook Definition:

Much Faster Than Average Job Outlook is when projected percent change in employment from 2021 to 2031 is much faster than the average growth rate for all occupations which is 5 percent.

CAREERS BY JOB OUTLOOK

Faster Than Average Growth (8-15%)

- **Audiologists**
- **Biological Technicians**
- **Biomedical Engineers**
- **Biochemists and Biophysicists**
- **Chiropractors**
- **Community Health Workers**
- **Dental Assistants**
- **Dental Hygienists**
- **Diagnostic Medical Sonographers**
- **Exercise Physiologists**
- **Health Education Specialists**
- **Occupational Therapists**
- **Optometrists**
- **Phlebotomists**
- **Psychiatric Technicians**
- **Rehabilitation Counselors**
- **Respiratory Therapists**
- **Social Workers**

Job Outlook Definition:

Faster Than Average Job Outlook is when projected percent change in employment from 2021 to 2031 is much faster than the average growth rate for all occupations which is 5 percent.

CAREERS BY JOB OUTOOK

Average Growth (4 - 7%)

- **Cardiovascular Technologists and Technicians**
- **Clinical Laboratory Technologists and Technicians**
- **Dentists**
- **Dietitian Nutritionists**
- **Emergency Medical Technician and Paramedics**
- **Licensed Practical and Licensed Vocational Nurses**
- **Medical Records Specialists**
- **MRI Technologists**
- **Nursing Assistants**
- **Opticians**
- **Pharmacy Technicians**
- **Radiation Therapists**
- **Radiologic Technologists**
- **Registered Nurses**
- **Surgical Technologists**
- **Wholesale and Manufacturing Sales Representatives**

Slower Than Average Growth (<3%)

- **Dental and Ophthalmic Laboratory Technicians and Medical Appliance Technicians**
- **Medical Transcriptionists**
- **Nuclear Medicine Technologists**
- **Pharmacists**
- **Physicians and Surgeons**
- **Podiatrists**

Job Outlook Definition:

Average Outlook is when projected percent change in employment from 2021 to 2031 is approximately the same as the average growth rate for all occupations which is 5 percent.

Slower Than Average is when projected percent change in employment from 2021 to 2031 is slower than the average growth rate for all occupations which is 5 percent.

CAREERS BY AVERAGE SALARY

Average Salary $25k-$49k

- **Athletic Trainers**
- **Biological Technicians**
- **Community Health Workers**
- **Dental and Ophthalmic Laboratory Technicians and Medical Appliance Technicians**
- **Dental Assistants**
- **Emergency Medical Technician and Paramedics**
- **Estheticians and Skincare Specialists**
- **Exercise Physiologists**
- **Health Education Specialists**
- **Home Health and Personal Care Aides**
- **Licensed Practical and Licensed Vocational Nurses**
- **Massage Therapists**
- **Medical Assistants**
- **Medical Records Specialists**
- **Medical Transcriptionists**
- **Nursing Assistants**
- **Opticians**
- **Pharmacy Technicians**
- **Phlebotomists**
- **Physical Therapist Assistants**
- **Psychiatric Technicians**
- **Rehabilitation Counselors**
- **Surgical Technologists**
- **Veterinary Technologists and Technicians**
- **Veterinary Assistants and Laboratory Animal Caretakers**

Average Salary $50k-$74k

- **Art Therapists**
- **Cardiovascular Technologists and Technicians**
- **Clinical Laboratory Technologists and Technicians**
- **Dietitian Nutritionists**
- **Health Information Technologists and Medical Registrars**
- **MRI Technologists**
- **Music Therapists**
- **Occupational Therapy Assistants**
- **Radiologic Technologists**
- **Respiratory Therapists**
- **Social Workers**
- **Wholesale and Manufacturing Sales Representatives**

CAREERS BY AVERAGE SALARY

Average Salary $75k-$99k

- Audiologists
- Biomedical Engineers
- Chiropractors
- Dental Hygienists
- Diagnostic Medical Sonographers
- Epidemiologists
- Medical Scientists
- Nuclear Medicine Technologists
- Occupational Therapists
- Orthotists and Prosthetists
- Physical Therapists
- Radiation Therapists
- Registered Nurses
- Speech Language Pathologists

Average Salary $100k+

- Biochemists and Biophysicists
- Dentists
- Medical and Health Services Managers
- Nurse Anesthetists
- Nurse Midwives
- Nurse Practitioners
- Optometrists
- Pharmacists
- Physicians and Surgeons
- Physician Assistants
- Podiatrists
- Veterinarians

ART THERAPISTS

OVERVIEW

Art therapists use art and psychology to help influence people and help people meet their goals through diverse art media and techniques. Art therapists help people reflect on their art, understand themselves, and process various thoughts and feelings.

Art therapy uses the creative process, making art, and applying psychological theory within a psychotherapeutic relationship to enrich the lives of individuals, families, and communities.

Art therapists typically do the following:

- Talk with clients about symptoms, medical history, and treatment goals
- Evaluate clients prior to and during the art therapy
- Discuss art media and techniques with clients
- Help client's implement creative skills and techniques
- Provide guidance on self reflection and processing thoughts and feelings
- Document clients' conditions and progress

Education Level

Master's Degree

Type of Area

Clinical

License or Certification

- Depends on State

Average Salary: $71k*	Number of Jobs in 2022: 16,920*
Average Hourly: $34/hr*	Job Outlook in 2021: N/A
Salary Range: $37k to $111k*	10y Change 2021 - 2031: N/A

Education Requirements

- Bachelor's Degree (4 years)
- Master's Degree (2 years)

Work Environment*

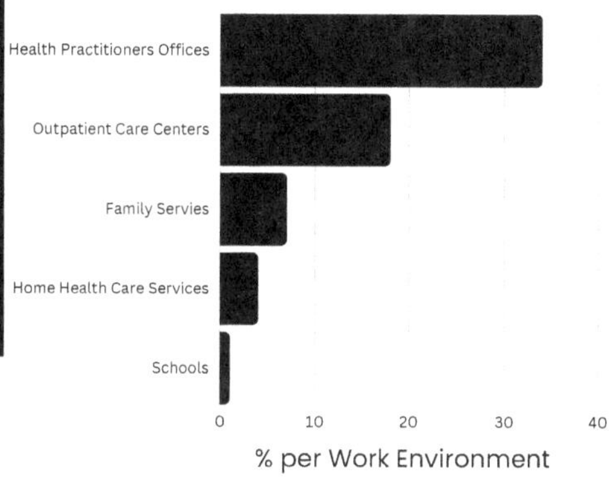

Resources:

- American Art Therapy Association: https://arttherapy.org/

*Data from Therapists, All Other

Source: U.S. BUREAU OF LABOR STATISTICS

ATHLETIC TRAINERS

OVERVIEW

Athletic trainers specialize in preventing, diagnosing, and treating muscle and bone injuries and illnesses for people of all ages.

Athletic trainers provide care when injuries occur on the field or during athletic events. They work with other healthcare providers to discuss injuries and treatment options or evaluate and treat patients.

Athletic trainers typically do the following:

- Apply protective or injury-preventive devices, such as tape, bandages, and braces
- Recognize and evaluate injuries
- Provide first aid or emergency care
- Develop and carry out rehabilitation programs for injured athletes
- Plan and implement comprehensive programs to prevent injury and illness among athletes

Education Level

Master's Degree

Type of Area

Clinical

License or Certification

- Depends on State

Average Salary: $48k	Number of Jobs in 2021: 29,400
Average Hourly: $23/hr	Job Outlook in 2021: 17%
Salary Range: $36k to $76k	10y Change 2021 - 2031: 5,100

Education Requirements

- Bachelor's degree (4 years)
- Master's Degree (2 years)

Work Environment

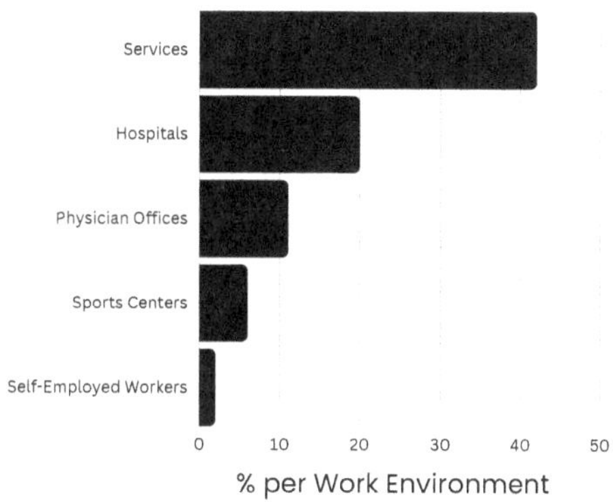

Resources:
- Commission on Accreditation of Athletic Training Education (CAATE): https://caate.net/

Source: U.S. BUREAU OF LABOR STATISTICS

AUDIOLOGISTS

OVERVIEW

Audiologists diagnose, manage, and treat patients who have hearing, balance, or related problems.

Audiologists use a variety of devices like audiometers to identify the extent and underlying cause of problems like hearing loss.

Audiologists' ability to diagnose as well as treat patients distinguishes their work from that of hearing aid specialists.

Audiologists typically do the following:

- Examine patients outer, middle, or inner ear problems
- Assess the results of the examination and diagnose problems
- Create and modify treatment plans to meet patients' goals
- Fit and dispense hearing aids and other assistive listening devices
- Counsel patients and their families on ways to listen and communicate
- Research the causes and treatment of hearing and balance disorders
- Educate patients on ways to prevent hearing loss

Education Level

Doctorate Degree

Type of Area

Clinical

License or Certification

- State License

Average Salary: $78k	Number of Jobs in 2021: 14,600
Average Hourly: **$38/hr**	**Job Outlook in 2021:** **10%**
Salary Range: **$58k to $120k**	**10y Change 2021 - 2031:** **1,500**

Work Environment

Education Requirements

- Bachelor's degree (4 years)
- Doctor of Audiology (4 years, Au.D)

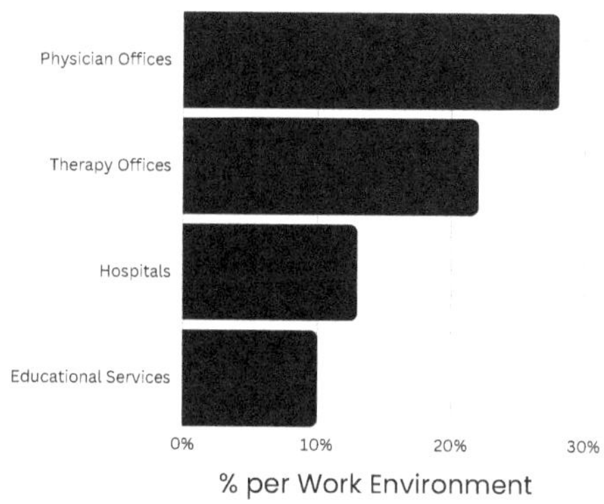

Resources:

- American Speech-Language-Hearing Association: http://www.asha.org/
- American Board of Audiology: https://www.audiology.org/american-board-of-audiology/

Source: U.S. BUREAU OF LABOR STATISTICS

BIOCHEMISTS AND BIOPHYSICISTS

OVERVIEW

Biochemists and biophysicists study the chemical and physical principles of living things and of biological processes, such as cell development, growth, heredity, and disease.

Biochemists and biophysicists use advanced technologies, such as lasers and fluorescent microscopes, to conduct scientific experiments and analyses.

Biochemists and biophysicists work in basic and applied research. Basic research is conducted without any immediately known application; the goal is to expand human knowledge. Applied research is directed toward solving a particular problem.

Biochemists and Biophysicists typically do the following:

- Plan and conduct complex projects in basic and applied research
- Manage laboratory teams
- Isolate, analyze, and synthesize proteins, fats, DNA, and other molecules
- Research the effects of substances such as drugs, hormones, and nutrients on tissues and biological processes
- Prepare technical reports, research papers, and recommendations based on their research findings

Education Level

Doctorate Degree

Type of Area

Clinical

License or Certification

- None

Average Salary:
$102k

Average Hourly:
$49/hr

Salary Range:
$61k to $167k

Number of Jobs in 2021:
37,500

Job Outlook in 2021:
15%

10y Change 2021 - 2031:
5,700

Education Requirements

- Bachelor's degree (4 years)
- Doctor of Philosophy (3+ years, PhD)
- Post-Doctoral Research

Work Environment

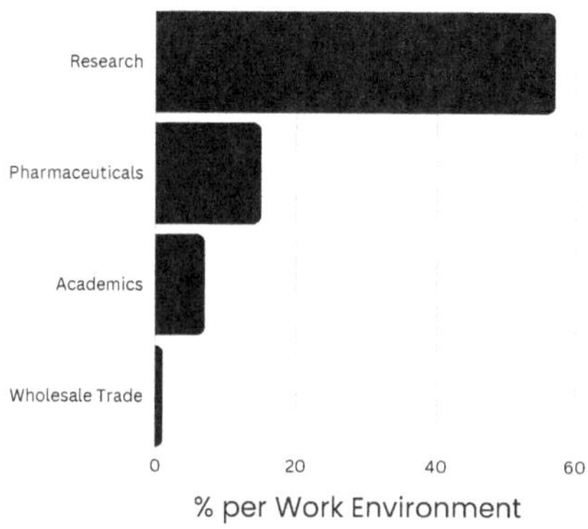

Resources:

- American Society for Biochemistry and Molecular Biology: https://www.asbmb.org/

Source: U.S. BUREAU OF LABOR STATISTICS

BIOLOGICAL TECHNICIANS

OVERVIEW

Biological technicians help biological and medical scientists conduct laboratory tests and experiments.

Biological technicians work in many research areas. They may assist medical researchers by administering new medicines and treatments to laboratory animals, if needed.

Biological technicians also may work in private industry and assist in the study of a wide range of topics concerning industrial production

Biological technicians typically do the following:

- Set up, maintain, and clean laboratory instruments and equipment, such as microscopes, scales, pipets, and test tubes
- Gather and prepare biological samples, such as blood, food, and bacteria cultures, for laboratory analysis
- Conduct biological tests and experiments
- Document their work, including procedures, observations, and results
- Analyze experimental data and interpret results
- Write reports that summarize their findings

Education Level

Bachelor's Degree

Type of Area

Non-Clinical

License or Certification

- None

Average Salary: $48k	**Number of Jobs in 2021:** 84,300
Average Hourly: $23/hr	**Job Outlook in 2021:** 9%
Salary Range: $31k to $78k	**10y Change 2021 - 2031:** 7,700

Education Requirements

- Bachelor's degree (4 years)

Work Environment

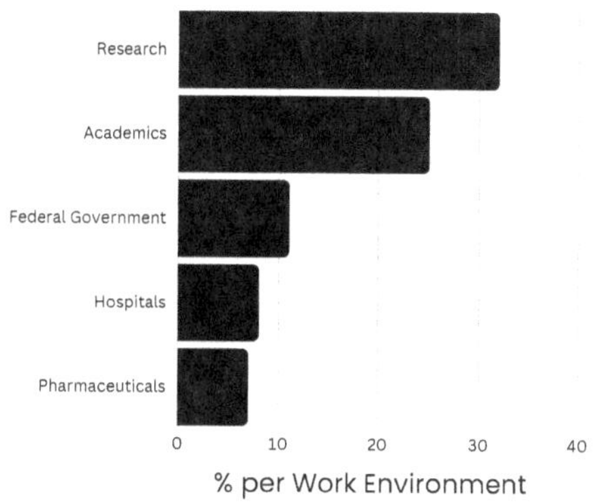

Source: U.S. BUREAU OF LABOR STATISTICS

BIOMEDICAL ENGINEERS

OVERVIEW

Biomedical engineers combine engineering principles with sciences to design and create equipment, devices, computer systems, and software.

Biomedical engineers focus on advances in technology and medicine to develop new devices and equipment for improving human health.

In addition, they design and build artificial body parts, such as hip and knee joints, or develop materials to make replacement parts.

Biomedical engineers typically do the following:

- Design equipment and devices, such as artificial internal organs and machines for diagnosing medical problems
- Install, maintain, or provide technical support for biomedical equipment
- Collaborate with manufacturing staff on the safety and effectiveness of biomedical equipment
- Train clinicians and others on the proper use of biomedical equipment
- Work with scientists to research how engineering principles apply to biological systems
- Develop statistical models or simulations
- Prepare procedures and write technical reports and research papers

Education Level

Bachelor's Degree

Type of Area

Non-Clinical

License or Certification

- None

Average Salary: **$97k**
Average Hourly: **$46/hr**
Salary Range: **$60k to $154k**

Number of Jobs in 2021: **17,900**
Job Outlook in 2021: **10%**
10y Change 2021 - 2031: **1,700**

Education Requirements

- Bachelor's degree (4 years)
- Graduate degree (2+ years), optional

Work Environment

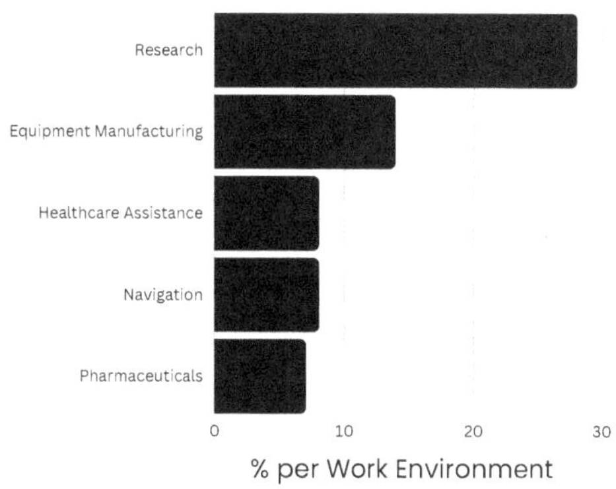

Note: Examples of types of bioengineers and biomedical engineers includes Biochemical engineers, Bioinstrumentation engineers, Biomaterials engineers, Biomechanics engineers, Clinical engineers, Genetic engineers, Rehabilitation engineers, and Systems physiologists.

Resources:

- American Institute for Medical and Biological Engineering: https://aimbe.org/
- Biomedical Engineering Society: https://www.bmes.org/

Source: U.S. BUREAU OF LABOR STATISTICS

CARDIOVASCULAR TECHNOLOGISTS AND TECHNICIANS

OVERVIEW

Cardiovascular technologists and technicians operate special equipment to create images or conduct tests.

They work closely with physicians and surgeons, who view the images and test results to assess and diagnose medical conditions.

Cardiovascular technologists and technicians create images and conduct tests involving the heart and lungs.

Cardiovascular technologists and technicians typically do the following:

- Prepare patients by explaining the procedure and answering questions
- Prepare exam rooms and maintain diagnostic imaging equipment
- Properly situate patients for imaging
- Operate equipment to obtain diagnostic images or to conduct tests
- Review images or test results to check for quality and adequate coverage of the areas needed for diagnoses
- Analyze results for abnormalities and other diagnostic information and provide a summary of findings to physicians
- Record findings and keep track of patients' records

Education Level

Associate's Degree

Type of Area

Clinical

License or Certification

- Depends on Employment

Average Salary: **$77k**
Average Hourly: **$29/hr**
Salary Range: **$59k to $101k**

Number of Jobs in 2021: **74,700**
Job Outlook in 2021: **7%**
10y Change 2021 - 2031: **5,100**

Work Environment

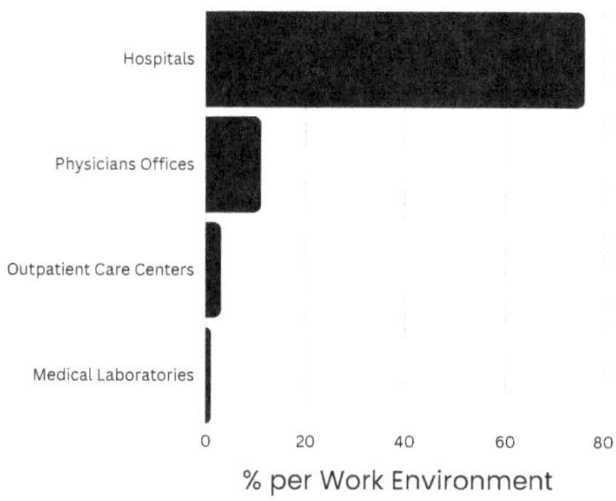

Education Requirements

- Associate's Degree (2 years)

Note: Examples of types of cardiovascular technologists and technicians includes Cardiovascular invasive specialists, Cardiographic or electrocardiogram (EKG) technicians, and Pulmonary function technologists

Resources:

- American Registry of Radiologic Technologists: https://www.arrt.org/

Source: U.S. BUREAU OF LABOR STATISTICS

CHIROPRACTORS

OVERVIEW

Chiropractors evaluate and treat patients' neuromusculoskeletal system, which includes nerves, bones, muscles, ligaments, and tendons.

They use spinal adjustments and manipulation, as well as other clinical interventions, to manage patients' health concerns, such as back and neck pain.

Some chiropractors treat patients using procedures such as massage therapy, rehabilitative exercise, and electrical muscle stimulation in addition to spinal adjustments and manipulation.

They also may apply supports, such as braces or tape, to treat patients and relieve pain.

Chiropractors typically do the following:

- Review a patient's medical history and listen to their concerns
- Perform a physical examination to analyze the patient's posture, spine, and reflexes
- Provide neuromusculoskeletal therapy, which involves adjusting a patient's spinal column and other joints
- Give additional treatments, such as applying heat or cold to a patient's injured areas
- Advise patients on health and lifestyle issues, such as exercise and nutrition

Education Level

Doctorate Degree

Type of Area

Clinical

License or Certification

- State License
- National Board of Chiropra
  Examiners (NBCE) Exam

Average Salary: $75k	Number of Jobs in 2021: 53,200
Average Hourly: $36/hr	Job Outlook in 2021: 10%
Salary Range: $37k to $128k	10y Change 2021 - 2031: 5,600

Education Requirements

- Bachelor's degree (4 years)
- Doctor of Chiropractic (4-5 years, D.C)

Work Environment

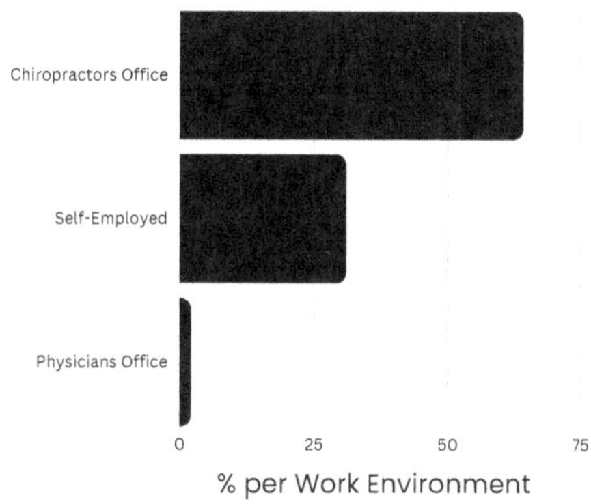

Note: In addition to operating a general chiropractic practice, chiropractors may specialize in areas such as sports, neurology, or nutrition.

Resources:

- American Chiropractic Association: https://www.acatoday.org/

Source: U.S. BUREAU OF LABOR STATISTICS

CLINICAL LABORATORY TECHNOLOGISTS AND TECHNICIANS

OVERVIEW

Clinical laboratory technologists (also known as medical laboratory technologists) and clinical laboratory technicians (also known as medical laboratory technicians) perform medical laboratory tests for the diagnosis, treatment, and prevention of disease.

Both technicians and technologists perform tests and procedures that physicians and surgeons or other healthcare practitioners order. However, technologists perform more complex tests and laboratory procedures than technicians do.

Clinical laboratory technologists and technicians set up, calibrate, and maintain the microscopes, cell counters, and other equipment they use.

Clinical laboratory technologists and technicians typically do the following:

- Test and analyze body fluids, such as blood, urine, and tissue samples
- Operate laboratory equipment, such as microscopes and automated cell counters
- Record data from medical tests and enter results into a patient's medical record
- Discuss results and findings of laboratory tests and procedures with physicians

Bachelor's Degree

Type of Area

Clinical

License or Certification

- Depends on State

Average Salary: $57k	Number of Jobs in 2021: 329,200
Average Hourly: $27/hr	Job Outlook in 2021: 7%
Salary Range: $30k to $79k	10y Change 2021 - 2031: 21,800

Education Requirements

- Bachelor's degree (4 years)

Work Environment

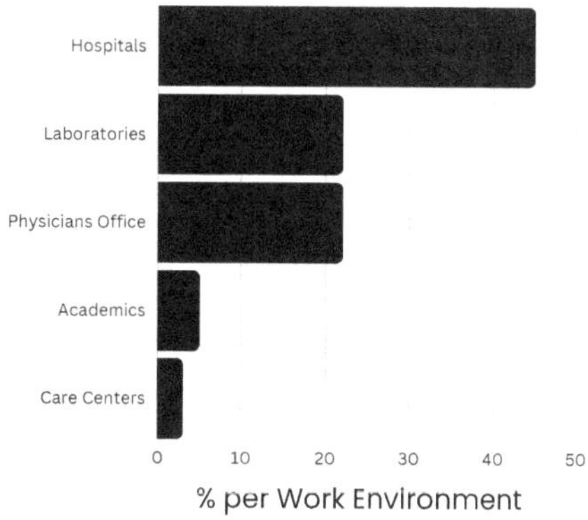

Note: Examples of types of specialized clinical laboratory technologists include Blood bank technologists, Clinical chemistry technologists, Cytotechnologists, Hematology technologists, Histotechnologists, Microbiology technologists, and Molecular biology technologists.

Resources:

- American Association of Bioanalysts: https://www.aab.org/
- American Medical Technologists: http://www.americanmedtech.org/
- American Society for Clinical Pathology: https://www.ascp.org/

Source: U.S. BUREAU OF LABOR STATISTICS

COMMUNITY HEALTH WORKERS

OVERVIEW

Community health workers advocate for residents' needs with healthcare providers and social service organizations. They implement wellness strategies by collecting data and discussing health concerns with members of specific populations.

Community health workers understand the communities they serve, which allows them to act as intermediaries between residents and healthcare and social services providers. They identify health-related issues, collect data, and discuss health concerns within the community.

Community health workers typically do the following:

- Discuss health concerns with community members
- Educate people about the importance and availability of healthcare services, such as cancer screenings
- Provide basic health services such as first aid, diabetic foot checks, and height and weight measurements
- Collect data to help identify community needs
- Report findings to health education specialists, healthcare workers, or social service providers
- Provide informal counseling and social support
- Conduct outreach programs
- Make referrals, provide transportation, and address other barriers to healthcare access
- Advocate for individual and community needs

Education Level

High School Diploma

Type of Area

Clinical

License or Certification

- Depends on State

Average Salary: **$46k**	**Number of Jobs in 2021:** **67,000**
Average Hourly: **$22/hr**	**Job Outlook in 2021:** **16%**
Salary Range: **$30k to $70k**	**10y Change 2021 - 2031:** **10,600**

Work Environment

Education Requirements

- On the Job Training

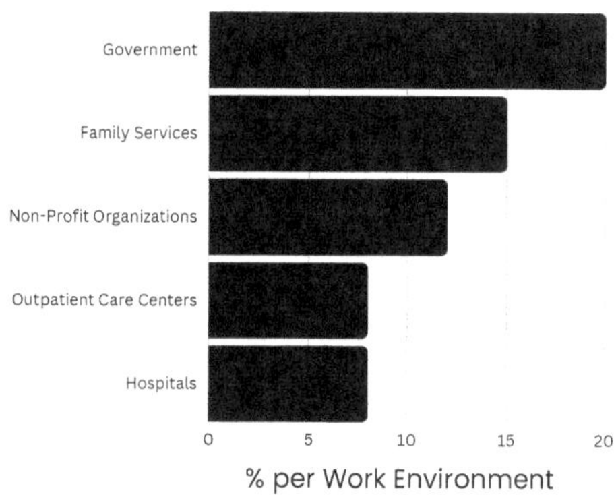

Resources:

- National Association of Community Health Workers: https://nachw.org/

Source: U.S. BUREAU OF LABOR STATISTICS

DENTAL AND OPHTHALMIC LABORATORY TECHNICIANS AND MEDICAL APPLIANCE TECHNICIANS

OVERVIEW

Dental and ophthalmic laboratory technicians and medical appliance technicians make or repair dentures, eyeglasses, prosthetics, and related products.

In small offices and retail establishments, technicians may handle every phase of production. In large manufacturing and wholesale facilities, technicians may be responsible for only one phase of production, such as polishing, measuring, or testing.

- Dental laboratory technicians use impressions or molds of a patient's teeth to create crowns, bridges, dentures, and other dental appliances.
- Ophthalmic laboratory technicians make prescription eyeglasses and contact lenses.
- Medical appliance technicians construct and repair medical supportive devices, such as hearing aids or leg braces.

Dental and Ophthalmic laboratory technicians and Medical appliance technicians typically do the following:

- Bend, form, and shape material for appliances or devices
- Polish and shape appliances and devices, using handtools or power tools
- Adjust appliances or devices to allow for a natural look or to improve function
- Repair damaged appliances and devices

Education Level

High School Diploma

Type of Area

Non-Clinical

License or Certification

- None

Average Salary: $39k
Average Hourly: $18/hr
Salary Range: $29k to $62k

Number of Jobs in 2021: 73,300
Job Outlook in 2021: 2%
10y Change 2021 - 2031: 1,400

Education Requirements

- On the Job Training

Work Environment

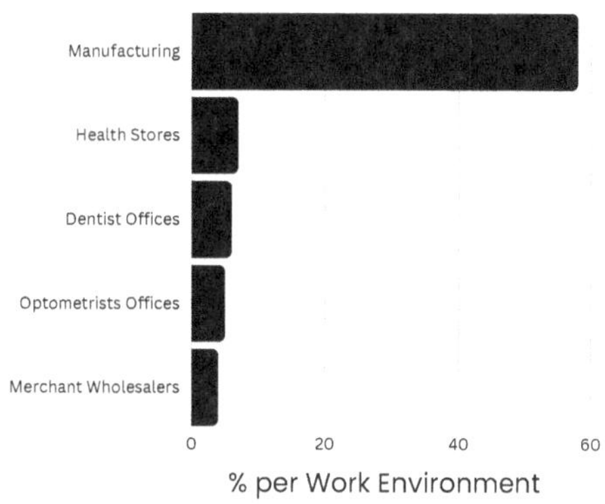

Resources:

- National Board for Certification in Dental Laboratory Technology: https://nbccert.org/
- American Board for Certification in Orthotics, Prosthetics & Pedorthics: https://www.ardms.org/

Source: U.S. BUREAU OF LABOR STATISTICS

DENTAL ASSISTANTS

OVERVIEW

Dental assistants work closely with patients and dentists helping with patient care, record-keeping, and appointment scheduling. Their duties vary by state and by the dentists' offices in which they work.

Dental assistants have a variety of tasks that range from helping take a patient's medical history and vitals, patient education, and assisting during dental procedures.

Dental assistants typically do the following:

- Ensure that patients are comfortable in the dental chair
- Prepare patients and the work area for treatments and procedures
- Sterilize dental instruments
- Hand instruments to dentists during procedures
- Dry patients' mouths using suction hoses and other equipment
- Instruct patients in proper oral hygiene
- Process x-rays and complete lab tasks, under the direction of a dentist
- Keep records of dental treatments
- Schedule patient appointments
- Work with patients on billing and payment

Education Level

Postsecondary Non-Degree

Type of Area

Clinical

License or Certification

- Depends on State

Average Salary: $38k	Number of Jobs in 2021: 358,600
Average Hourly: $18/hr	Job Outlook in 2021: 8%
Salary Range: $29k to $59k	10y Change 2021 - 2031: 30,100

Education Requirements

- Accredited Program or
- On the Job Training

Work Environment

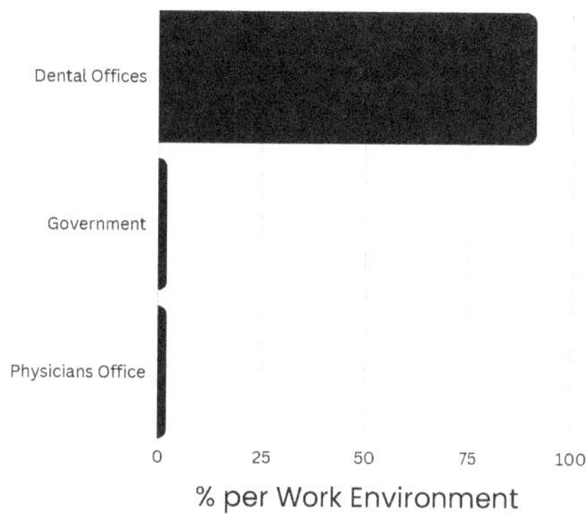

Resources:

- American Dental Assistants Association: https://www.adaausa.org/

Source: U.S. BUREAU OF LABOR STATISTICS

DENTAL HYGIENISTS

OVERVIEW

Dental hygienists examine patients for signs of oral diseases, such as gingivitis, and provide preventive care, including oral hygiene. They also educate patients about oral health.

Dental hygienists use many types of tools like hand, power, and ultrasonic tools. Hygienists remove stains with an air-polishing device and polish teeth with a power tool. Hygienists also use x-ray machines to take pictures to check for tooth or jaw problems.

Dental hygienists typically do the following:

- Remove tartar, stains, and plaque from teeth
- Apply sealants and fluorides to help protect teeth
- Take and develop dental x-rays
- Assess patients' oral health and report findings to dentists
- Document patient care and treatment plans
- Educate patients about oral hygiene techniques, such as how to brush and floss correctly

Education Level

Associate's Degree

Type of Area

Clinical

License or Certification

- State License

Average Salary: $77k	Number of Jobs in 2021: 214,000
Average Hourly: $37/hr	Job Outlook in 2021: 9%
Salary Range: $60k to $100k	10y Change 2021 - 2031: 19,000

Education Requirements

- Associate's Degree (3 years)
- Bachelor's Degree (4 years)

Work Environment

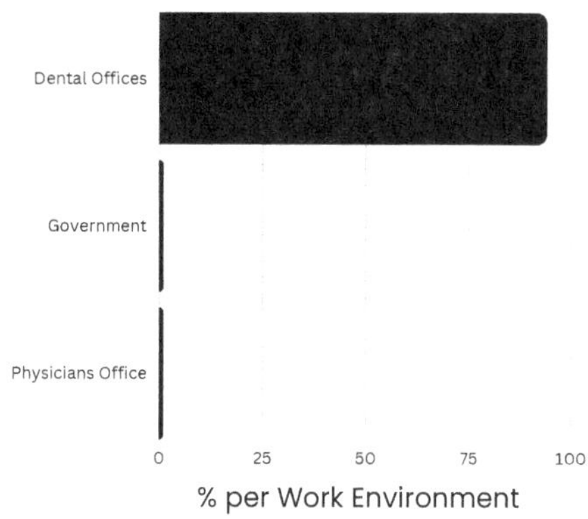

Resources:

- American Dental Hygienists' Association: https://www.adha.org/

Source: U.S. BUREAU OF LABOR STATISTICS

DENTISTS

OVERVIEW

Dentists diagnose and treat problems with patients' teeth, gums, and related parts of the mouth. They provide advice and instruction on taking care of the teeth and gums and on diet choices that affect oral health.

Dentists use a variety of equipment, including x-ray machines, drills, mouth mirrors, probes, forceps, brushes, and scalpels. They also use lasers, digital scanners, and other technologies.

***Dentists typically do the following*:**

- Remove decay from teeth and fill cavities
- Repair or remove damaged teeth
- Place sealants or whitening agents on teeth
- Administer anesthetics to keep patients from feeling pain during procedures
- Prescribe antibiotics or other medications
- Examine x-rays of teeth, gums, the jaw, and nearby areas in order to diagnose problems
- Make models and measurements for dental appliances, such as dentures
- Teach patients about diets, flossing, the use of fluoride, and other aspects of dental care

Education Level

Doctorate Degree

Type of Area

Clinical

License or Certification

- State License
- National Board Dental Examination

Average Salary: **$163k**	**Number of Jobs in 2021:** **146,200**
Average Hourly: **$78/hr**	**Job Outlook in 2021:** **6%**
Salary Range: **$63k to $208k**	**10y Change 2021 - 2031:** **8,400**

Education Requirements

- Bachelor's Degree (4 years)
- Doctor of Dental Surgery (DDS) or Doctor of Medicine in Dentistry (DMD) (4 years)
- Residency, if specializing

Work Environment

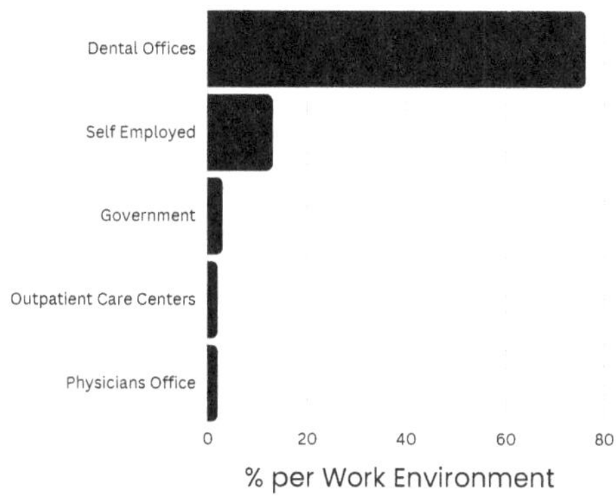

Note: Some dentists practice in a specialty area like Dental anesthesiologists, Dental public health specialists, Endodontists, Oral and maxillofacial radiologists, Oral and maxillofacial surgeons, Oral pathologists, Orthodontists, Pediatric dentists, and Periodontists.

Resources:

- American Dental Association: https://www.ada.org/

Source: U.S. BUREAU OF LABOR STATISTICS

DIAGNOSTIC MEDICAL SONOGRAPHERS

OVERVIEW

Diagnostic medical sonographers operate special equipment to create images or conduct tests. They work closely with physicians and surgeons, who view the images and test results to assess and diagnose medical conditions.

Diagnostic medical sonographers specialize in creating images, known as sonograms or ultrasounds, that depict the body's organs and tissues. Sonography uses sound waves to produce images and is often the first imaging test performed when disease is suspected.

Diagnostic medical sonographers typically do the following:

- Prepare patients by explaining the procedure and answering questions
- Prepare exam rooms and maintain diagnostic imaging equipment
- Properly situate patients for imaging
- Operate equipment to obtain diagnostic images or to conduct tests
- Review images or test results to check for quality and adequate coverage of the areas needed for diagnoses
- Analyze results for abnormalities and other diagnostic information and provide a summary of findings to physicians
- Record findings and keep track of patients' records

Education Level

Associate's Degree

Type of Area

Clinical

License or Certification

- Depends on Employment

Average Salary:
$60k

Average Hourly:
$28/hr

Salary Range:
$29k to $98k

Number of Jobs in 2021:
58,100

Job Outlook in 2021:
5%

10y Change 2021 - 2031:
2,700

Education Requirements

- Associate's Degree (2 years)

Work Environment

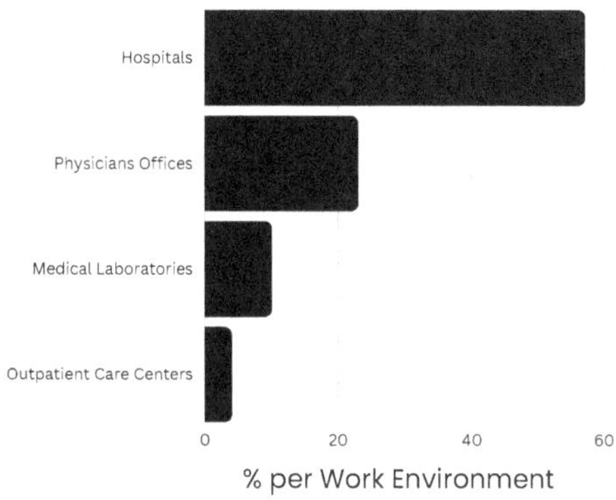

Note: Examples of types of medical sonographers include Abdominal sonographers, Breast sonographers, Cardiac sonographers (echocardiographers), Musculoskeletal sonographers, Obstetric and gynecologic sonographers, and Vascular technologists (vascular sonographers).

Resources:

- American Registry for Diagnostic Medical Sonographers: https://www.ardms.org/
- Society of Diagnostic Medical Sonography: https://www.sdms.org/

Source: U.S. BUREAU OF LABOR STATISTICS

DIETITIAN AND NUTRITIONISTS

OVERVIEW

Dietitians and nutritionists are experts in the use of food and nutrition to promote health and manage disease. They plan and conduct food service or nutritional programs to help people lead healthy lives.

Dietitians and nutritionists utilize nutrition assessment and diagnostic laboratory testing to evaluate clients. They advise clients on behavior modifications and intervention plans, including which foods to eat or avoid to improve their health.

Dietitians and nutritionists help prevent or support treatment of health conditions such as heart disease, autoimmune disease, and obesity.

Dietitian nutritionists typically do the following:

- Assess clients' nutritional and health needs
- Counsel clients on nutrition issues and healthy eating habits
- Develop meal and nutrition plans, taking clients' preferences and budgets into account
- Evaluate and monitor the effects of nutrition plans and practices
- Promote healthy lifestyles by speaking to groups about diet, nutrition, and the relationship between good eating habits and preventing or managing specific diseases
- Keep up with or contribute to the latest food and nutritional science research

Education Level

Bachelor's Degree

Type of Area

Clinical

License or Certification

- Depends on State

Average Salary:
$61k

Average Hourly:
$29/hr

Salary Range:
$42k to $93k

Number of Jobs in 2021:
74,700

Job Outlook in 2021:
7%

10y Change 2021 - 2031:
5,100

Education Requirements

- Bachelor's Degree (4 years)
- Internship Training (8-24 months)

Work Environment

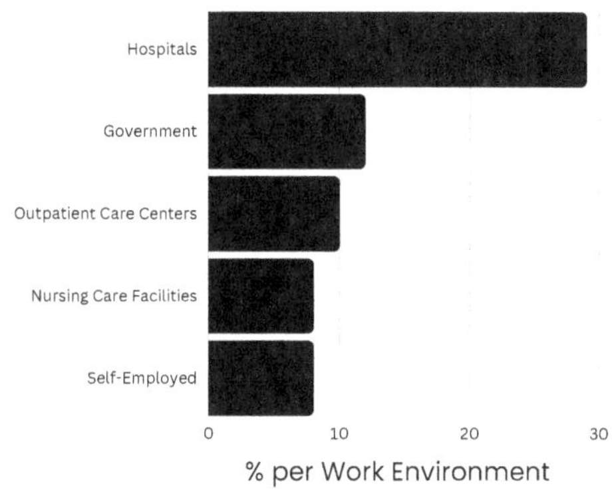

Resources:

- Academy of Nutrition and Dietetics: http://www.eatright.org/

Source: U.S. BUREAU OF LABOR STATISTICS

EMERGENCY MEDICAL TECHNICIANS AND PARAMEDICS

OVERVIEW

Emergency medical technicians (EMTs) and paramedics assess injuries and illnesses, provide emergency medical care, and may transport patients to medical facilities.

When transporting a patient in an ambulance, one EMT or paramedic may drive the ambulance while another monitors the patient's vital signs and provides emergency medical care. Some paramedics work as part of a helicopter's or an airplane's flight crew to transport critically ill or injured patients to a hospital.

In addition to transporting patients from the scene of an emergency, EMTs and paramedics transfer patients from one medical facility to another.

EMTs and Paramedics typically do the following:

- Respond to calls for medical assistance, such as at the scene of a car accident
- Assess people's condition and determine what treatment, if any, is needed
- Provide treatment, such as first aid or life support care, to sick or injured patients
- Prepare patients for and safely transport them to the emergency department of a hospital or other healthcare facility
- Document and report observations and any treatment provided, to physicians, nurses, or other healthcare staff

Education Level

Postsecondary Non-Degree

Type of Area

Clinical

License or Certification

- State License
- National Registry of Emerg
  Medical Technicians (NREM

Average Salary: **$36k**	**Number of Jobs in 2021:** **261,000**
Average Hourly: **$17/hr**	**Job Outlook in 2021:** **7%**
Salary Range: **$23k to $47k**	**10y Change 2021 - 2031:** **17,900**

Education Requirements

- Education Program (1-2 years)

Work Environment

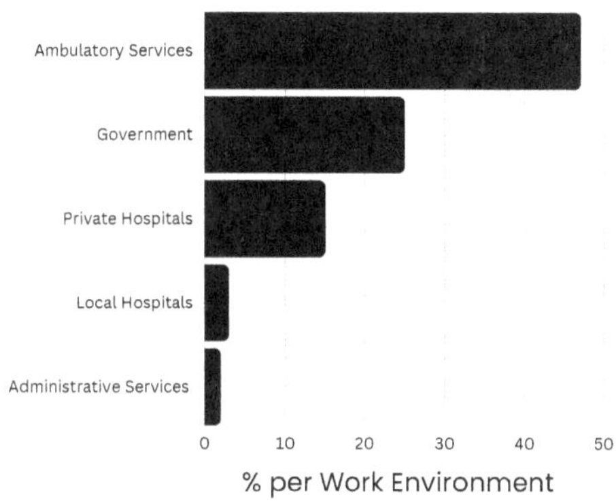

Note: The specific responsibilities of EMTs and paramedics depend on their level of certification and the state in which they work. EMTs can be basic or advanced EMTs.

Resources:

- National Association of Emergency Medical Technicians: https://www.naemt.org/

Source: U.S. BUREAU OF LABOR STATISTICS

EPIDEMIOLOGISTS

OVERVIEW

Epidemiologists are public health workers who investigate patterns and causes of disease and injury. They seek to reduce the risk and occurrence of negative health outcomes through research, community education and health policy.

Epidemiologists collect and analyze data to investigate health issues. Epidemiologists typically work in applied public health or in research. Applied epidemiologists work for state and local governments, often addressing public health problems through education outreach and survey efforts in communities. Research epidemiologists typically work for universities or in affiliation with federal agencies, such as the CDC or NIH.

Epidemiologists typically do the following:

- Plan and direct studies of public health problems to find ways to prevent them or to treat them if they arise
- Collect and analyze information from observations, interviews, surveys, and blood samples to find the causes of diseases or other health problems
- Communicate findings to health practitioners, policymakers, and the public
- Manage programs through planning, monitoring progress, and seeking ways to improve
- Write grant proposals to fund research

Education Level

Master's Degree

Type of Area

Non-Clinical

License or Certification

- None

Average Salary: **$78k**	**Number of Jobs in 2021:** **8,600**
Average Hourly: **$37/hr**	**Job Outlook in 2021:** **26%**
Salary Range: **$50k to $130k**	**10y Change 2021 - 2031:** **2,200**

Education Requirements

- Bachelor's Degree (4 years)
- Master's Degree (2 years)

Work Environment

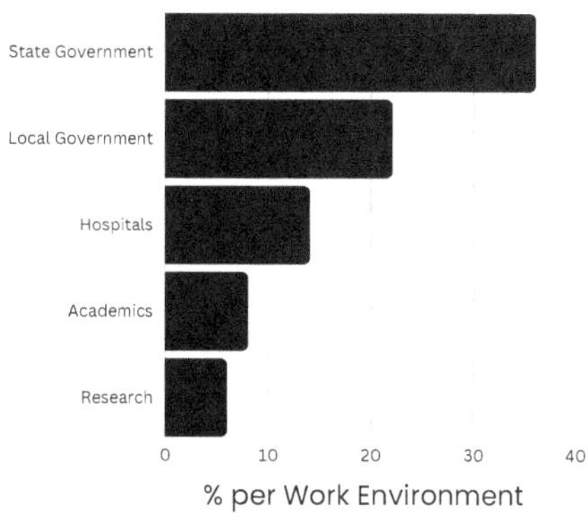

Note: Epidemiologists typically specialize in one or more public health areas, including the following Chronic diseases, Environmental health, Genetic and molecular epidemiology, Infectious diseases, Injury, Maternal and child health, Mental health, Public health preparedness and emergency response, and Veterinary epidemiology

Resources:

- American College of Epidemiology: https://www.acepidemiology.org/
- American Public Health Association: https://www.apha.org/

Source: U.S. BUREAU OF LABOR STATISTICS

ESTHETICIANS AND SKINCARE SPECIALISTS

OVERVIEW

Skincare specialists, also known as estheticians, provide cleansing and other face and body treatments to enhance a person's appearance.

Skincare specialists give facials, full-body treatments, and head and neck massages to improve the health and appearance of the skin. Some provide other skincare treatments to remove dead or dry skin, such as masks, peels, and scrubs. They also may provide eyelash services, makeup application, and hair removal.

In addition, these specialists create daily skincare routines for clients based on skin analysis and help them understand which products will work best for them.

Skincare specialists typically do the following:

- Evaluate clients' skin condition and appearance
- Discuss available treatments and determine which products will improve clients' skin quality
- Remove unwanted hair, using wax, lasers, or other approved treatments
- Recommend skincare products, such as cleansers, creams, or lotions
- Teach and advise clients on how to apply makeup and how to care for their skin
- Refer clients to another skincare specialist, such as a dermatologist, for serious skin problems

Education Level

Postsecondary Non-Degree

Type of Area

Clinical

License or Certification

- State License

Average Salary: $37k	**Number of Jobs in 2021:** 80,500
Average Hourly: $17/hr	**Job Outlook in 2021:** 17%
Salary Range: $11/hr to $31/hr	**10y Change 2021 - 2031:** 13,400

Education Requirements

- Education Program (4-6 months)

Work Environment

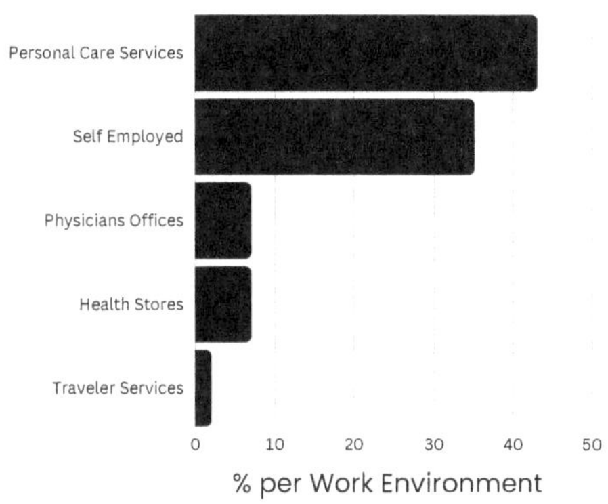

Resources:

- Associated Skin Care Professionals: https://www.ascpskincare.com/

Source: U.S. BUREAU OF LABOR STATISTICS

EXERCISE PHYSIOLOGISTS

OVERVIEW

Exercise physiologists develop fitness and exercise programs that help patients recover from chronic diseases and improve cardiovascular function, body composition, and flexibility.

Exercise physiologists work to improve overall patient health. Many of their patients suffer from health problems such as cardiovascular disease or pulmonary (lung) disease. Exercise physiologists provide health education and exercise plans to improve key health indicators.

Exercise physiologists typically do the following:

- Analyze a patient's medical history to assess their risk during exercise and to determine the best possible exercise and fitness regimen for the patient
- Perform fitness and stress tests with medical equipment and analyze the resulting patient data
- Measure blood pressure, oxygen usage, heart rhythm, and other key patient health indicators
- Develop exercise programs to improve patients' health

Education Level

Bachelor's Degree

Type of Area

Clinical

License or Certification

- None

Average Salary: **$47k**	**Number of Jobs in 2021:** **21,400**
Average Hourly: **$23/hr**	**Job Outlook in 2021:** **9%**
Salary Range: **$36k to $76k**	**10y Change 2021 - 2031:** **1,900**

Education Requirements

- Bachelor's Degree (4 years)

Work Environment

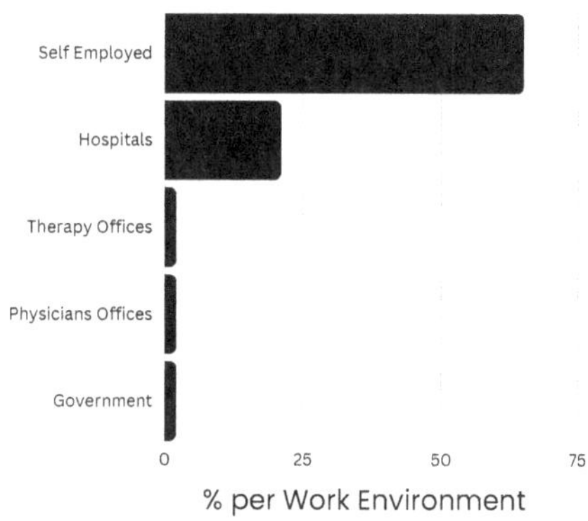

Resources:

- American Society of Exercise Physiologists: https://www.asep.org/

Source: U.S. BUREAU OF LABOR STATISTICS

HEALTH EDUCATION SPECIALISTS

OVERVIEW

Health education specialists teach people about behaviors that promote wellness. They develop strategies to improve the well-being of individuals and communities.

In healthcare facilities, health education specialists may work one-on-one with patients or their families. In nonprofits, health education specialists create programs and materials about health issues in the community they serve. In public health departments, health education specialists develop public health campaigns on topics such as emergency preparedness, immunizations, or proper nutrition.

Health education specialists typically do the following:

- Assess the health needs of individuals and communities
- Develop programs, materials, and events to teach people about health topics, such as managing existing conditions
- Evaluate the effectiveness of programs and educational materials
- Help people find health services or information
- Provide training programs for community health workers or other healthcare providers
- Supervise staff who implement health education programs
- Collect and analyze data to learn about a particular community and improve programs and services
- Advocate for improved health resources and policies that promote health

Education Level

Bachelor's Degree

Type of Area

Clinical

License or Certification

- Depends on State

Average Salary: $60k	Number of Jobs in 2021: 59,600
Average Hourly: $28/hr	Job Outlook in 2021: 8%
Salary Range: $37k to $102k	10y Change 2021 - 2031: 4,500

Education Requirements

- Bachelor's Degree (4 years)

Work Environment

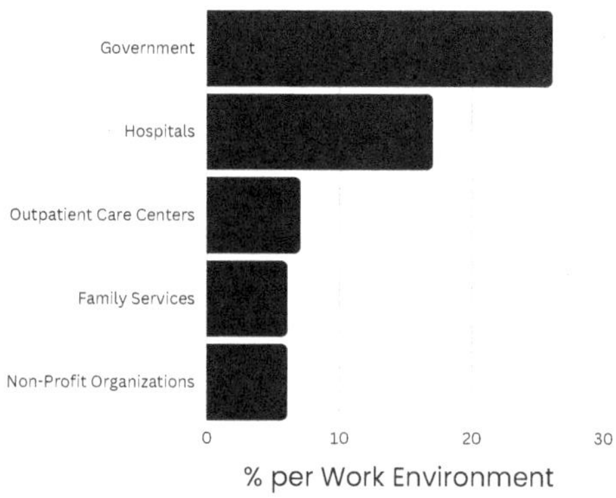

Resources:

- Society for Public Health Education: https://www.sophe.org/

Source: U.S. BUREAU OF LABOR STATISTICS

HEALTH INFORMATION TECHNOLOGISTS AND MEDICAL REGISTRARS

OVERVIEW

Health information technologists and medical registrars advise organizations on computerized healthcare systems and analyze clinical data.

Health information technologists apply their knowledge of information technology (IT) and healthcare concepts in a variety of ways. Some specialize in the electronic health records systems used for storing and retrieving patient data while others analyze healthcare data for a range of purposes, such as for research or to evaluate programs and services.

Medical registrars create and maintain databases of information, such as those used to track a particular disease or condition. They review patients' records and pathology reports to verify completeness and accuracy; assign classification codes to represent the diagnosis and treatment; and track treatment and outcomes.

Health information technologists and Medical registrars typically do the following:

- Help to determine requirements for computerized healthcare systems
- Evaluate and support implementation of health information systems
- Organize and update information in clinical databases or registries
- Compile data and generate reports, such as for disease registry or treatment
- Track patient outcomes for quality assessment
- Validate the integrity of patient data
- Ensure privacy, security, and confidentiality of patients' health information

Education Level

Associate's Degree

Type of Area

Non-Clinical

License or Certification

- None

Average Salary: **$55k**	**Number of Jobs in 2021:** **39,900**
Average Hourly: **$26/hr**	**Job Outlook in 2021:** **17%**
Salary Range: **$29k to $98k**	**10y Change 2021 - 2031:** **7,000**

Work Environment

Education Requirements

- Associate's Degree
- Bachelor's Degree (4 years), if applicable

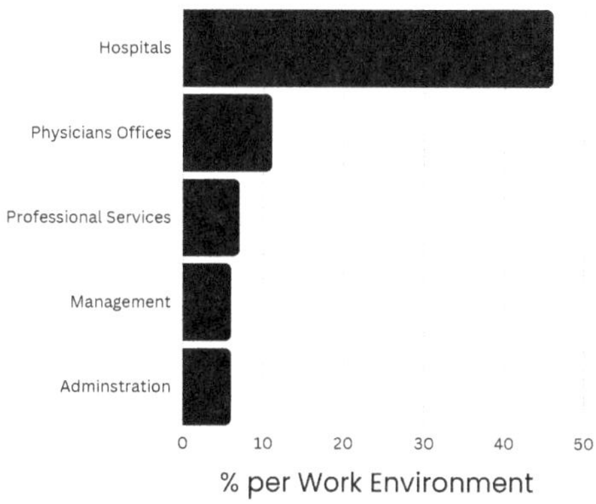

Note: Employers may prefer certifications. Credentials for a variety of specializations including the Registered Health Information Technician (RHIT), the Certified Documentation Improvement Practitioner (CDIP), and the Certified Health Data Analyst (CHDA).

Resources:

- American Health Information Management Association: https://www.ahima.org/

Source: U.S. BUREAU OF LABOR STATISTICS

HOME HEALTH AND PERSONAL CARE AIDS

OVERVIEW

Home health and personal care aides monitor the condition of people with disabilities or chronic illnesses and help them with daily living activities.

Under the direction of a nurse or other healthcare practitioner, home health aides may be allowed to give a client medication or to check the client's vital signs. Occasionally, they change bandages or dressings, give massages, care for skin, or help with braces and artificial limbs.

Personal care aides, sometimes called caregivers or personal attendants, are generally limited to providing non-medical services, including companionship, cleaning, cooking, and driving. Some of these aides work specifically with people who have developmental or intellectual disabilities to help create a behavior plan and teach self-care skills.

Home health and Personal care aides typically do the following:

- Assist clients in their daily personal tasks, such as bathing or dressing
- Perform housekeeping tasks, such as laundry and washing dishes
- Help to organize a client's schedule and plan appointments
- Arrange transportation to doctors' offices or other outings
- Shop for groceries and prepare meals to meet a client's dietary specifications
- Keep clients engaged in their social networks and communities

Education Level

High School Diploma

Type of Area

Clinical

License or Certification

- Depends on Employment

Average Salary: **$29k**	**Number of Jobs in 2021:** **3,636,900**
Average Hourly: **$14/hr**	**Job Outlook in 2021:** **25%**
Salary Range: **$22k to $37k**	**10y Change 2021 - 2031:** **924,000**

Education Requirements

- High School Diploma
- On the Job Training or Short Training Program

Work Environment

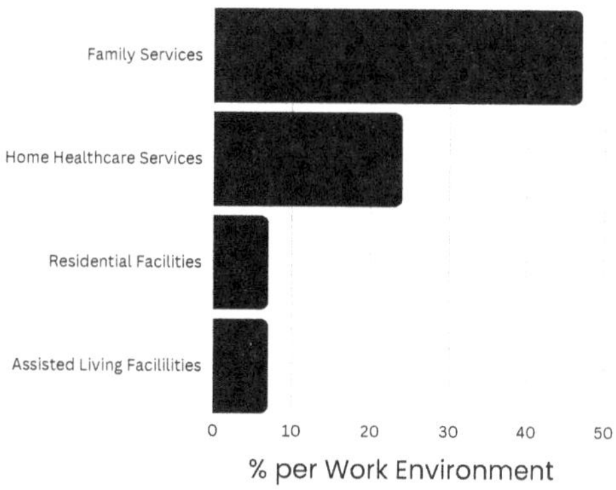

Source: U.S. BUREAU OF LABOR STATISTICS

LICENSED PRACTICAL AND VOCATIONAL NURSES

OVERVIEW

Licensed practical nurses (LPNs) and licensed vocational nurses (LVNs) provide basic medical care to ill or injured patients. Responsibilities for LPNs and LVNs are nearly identical; their title depends on the state in which they work.

Responsibilities of LPNs and LVNs vary by work setting. Some examples include providing patient education, collecting lab samples, and assisting patients with eating depending on the setting and needs.

Licensed Practical and Vocational Nurses typically do the following:

- Monitor patients' health by checking their vital signs
- Provide basic patient care and comfort, including changing bandages and helping with bathing
- Discuss care with patients and listen to their concerns
- Report patients' status and concerns to registered nurses, advanced practice nurses, or physicians
- Document patient care and maintain health records

Education Level

Postsecondary Non-Degree

Type of Area

Clinical

License or Certification

- State License
- National Council Licensure Examination (NCLEX-PN)

Average Salary: $48k	**Number of Jobs in 2021:** 657,200
Average Hourly: $23/hr	**Job Outlook in 2021:** 6%
Salary Range: $37k to $63k	**10y Change 2021 - 2031:** 41,300

Work Environment

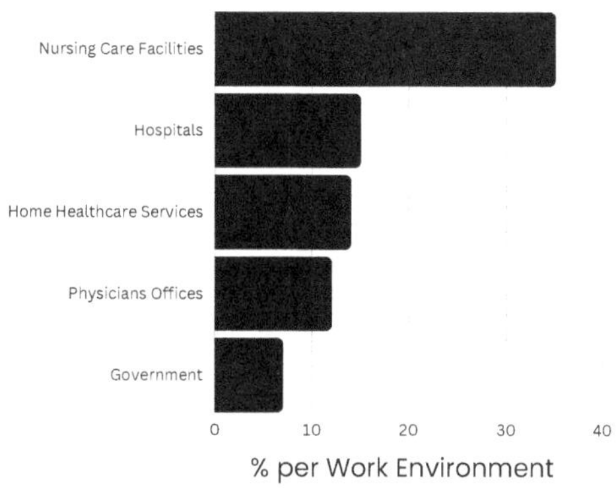

Education Requirements

- Education Program (1 year)

Resources:

- National Association of Licensed Practical Nurses: https://nalpn.org/
- American Nursing Association: https://www.nursingworld.org/

Source: U.S. BUREAU OF LABOR STATISTICS

MASSAGE THERAPISTS

OVERVIEW

Massage therapists treat clients by applying pressure to manipulate the body's soft tissues and joints. This treatment may help to relieve pain, heal injuries, relieve stress, and aid in the general wellness of clients.

Massage therapists manipulate clients' soft tissues and joints to treat injuries and promote general wellness. They may use their hands, fingers, forearms, elbows, and feet as tools during the session. Massage therapists may use lotions and oils and massage tables or chairs when treating a client. The length of a session varies based on type of massage.

Massage therapists talk with clients about what the desired outcome of massage and suggest personalized treatment plans for the client. They can specialize in different massage modalities, or specialties, such as Swedish massage, deep-tissue massage, and sports massage.

Massage Therapists typically do the following:

- Talk with clients about their symptoms, medical history, and treatment goals
- Evaluate clients prior to and during the massage to locate painful or tense areas of the body
- Manipulate muscles, tendons, ligaments, and other soft tissues of the body
- Increase range of motion through joint mobilization techniques
- Provide guidance on stretching, strengthening, overall relaxation, and improving their posture
- Document clients' conditions and progress

Education Level

Postsecondary Non-Degree

Type of Area

Clinical

License or Certification

- Depends on State
- Massage and Bodywork Licensing Examination (M

Average Salary: $46k
Average Hourly: $22/hr
Salary Range: $24k to $77k

Number of Jobs in 2021: 149,900
Job Outlook in 2021: 20%
10y Change 2021 - 2031: 29,900

Education Requirements

- Education Program (1-2 years)

Work Environment

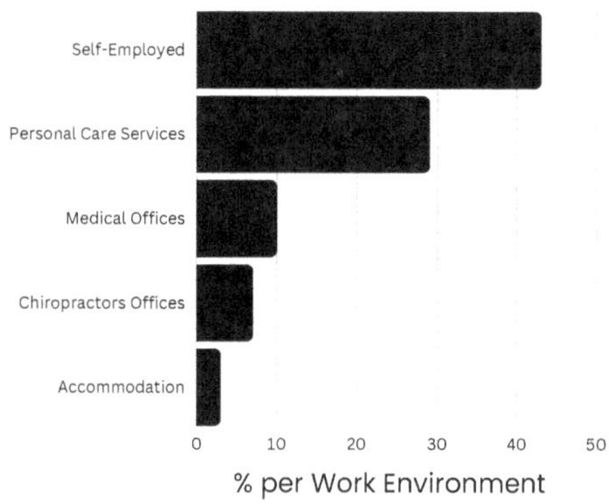

Resources:

- American Massage Therapy Association: https: //www.amtamassage.org/
- Associated Bodywork & Massage Professionals: http://www.abmp.com/

Source: U.S. BUREAU OF LABOR STATISTICS

MEDICAL AND HEALTH SERVICES MANAGERS

OVERVIEW

Medical and health services managers, also called healthcare executives or healthcare administrators, plan, direct, and coordinate medical and health services. They may manage an entire facility, a specific clinical area or department, or a medical practice for a group of physicians. Medical and health services managers must adapt to changes in healthcare laws, regulations, and technology.

Medical and health services managers set and carry out policies, goals, and procedures for their departments or facilities. Their duties include hiring, scheduling, and evaluating staff; monitoring compliance with state and federal guidelines; and developing reports and budgets. Responsibilities may vary by employer.

Medical and health services managers typically do the following:

- Develop goals and objectives related to efficiency and quality of healthcare services
- Ensure that the facility in which they work complies with laws and regulations
- Prepare and monitor budgets and manage finances, including patient fees and billing
- Recruit, train, and supervise staff members
- Represent the facility or department at investor meetings or on governing boards
- Keep and organize records of facility services, such as the number of inpatient beds used

Education Level

Bachelor's Degree

Type of Area

Non-Clinical

License or Certification

- Depends on Employment

Average Salary: $101k
Average Hourly: $48/hr
Salary Range: $60k to $205k

Number of Jobs in 2021: 480,700
Job Outlook in 2021: 28%
10y Change 2021 - 2031: 136,200

Education Requirements

- Bachelor's Degree (4 years)

Work Environment

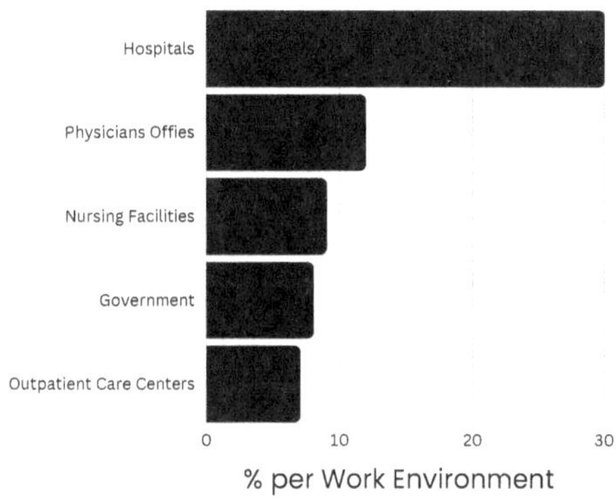

Note: Examples of types of Medical and Health Services Managers include Nursing home administrators, Clinical managers, and Health information managers.

Resources:

- American Association of Healthcare Administration Management: https://aaham.org/

Source: U.S. BUREAU OF LABOR STATISTICS

MEDICAL ASSISTANTS

OVERVIEW

Medical assistants complete administrative and clinical tasks in the offices of physicians, hospitals, and other healthcare facilities. Their duties vary with the location, specialty, and size of the practice.

Medical assistants take and record patients' personal information. They must be able to keep that information confidential and discuss it only with other medical personnel who are involved in treating the patient.

Medical assistants typically do the following:

- Record patient history and personal information
- Measure vital signs, such as blood pressure
- Help physicians with patient examinations
- Give patients injections or medications as directed by physicians and as permitted by state law
- Schedule patient appointments
- Prepare blood samples for laboratory tests
- Enter patient information into medical records

Education Level

Postsecondary Non-Degree

Type of Area

Clinical

License or Certification

- Depends on Employment

Average Salary: **$37k**	**Number of Jobs in 2021:** **743,500**
Average Hourly: **$17/hr**	**Job Outlook in 2021:** **16%**
Salary Range: **$29k to $48k**	**10y Change 2021 - 2031:** **117,800**

Education Requirements

- Education program (1 year) or On the Job Training

Work Environment

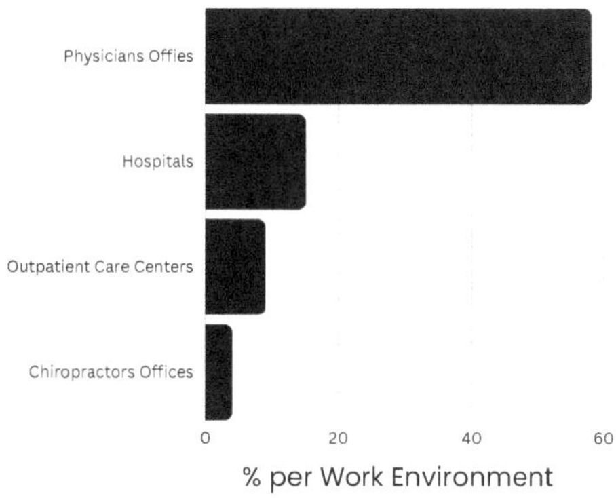

Note: Medical assistants should not be confused with physician assistants, who examine, diagnose, and treat patients under a physician's supervision. In larger practices or hospitals, medical assistants may specialize in either administrative or clinical work.

Resources:

- American Association of Medical Assistants: https://www.aama-ntl.org/

Source: U.S. BUREAU OF LABOR STATISTICS

MEDICAL RECORDS SPECIALISTS

OVERVIEW

Medical records specialists compile, process, and maintain patient files. They also may classify and enter patients' medical information into the healthcare industry's numerical coding system.

Medical records specialists have a variety of data entry and record-keeping tasks. They may gather patients' medical histories, symptoms, test results, treatments, and other health information and enter the details into electronic health records (EHR) systems. Some workers categorize medical information for purposes such as insurance reimbursement and providing data to clinicians.

Medical records specialists typically do the following:

- Review patients' records for timeliness, completeness, and accuracy
- Use classification systems to assign clinical codes for patients' diagnoses, procedures, medical services, and related information
- Maintain and retrieve records for insurance reimbursement and data analysis
- Electronically record data for collection, storage, analysis, retrieval, and reporting
- Ensure confidentiality of patients' records

Education Level

Postsecondary Non-Degree

Type of Area

Non-Clinical

License or Certification

- Depends on Employment

Average Salary: $46k	Number of Jobs in 2021: 186,400
Average Hourly: $22/hr	Job Outlook in 2021: 7%
Salary Range: $29k to $74k	10y Change 2021 - 2031: 12,300

Education Requirements

- Education program (1-2 years)

Work Environment

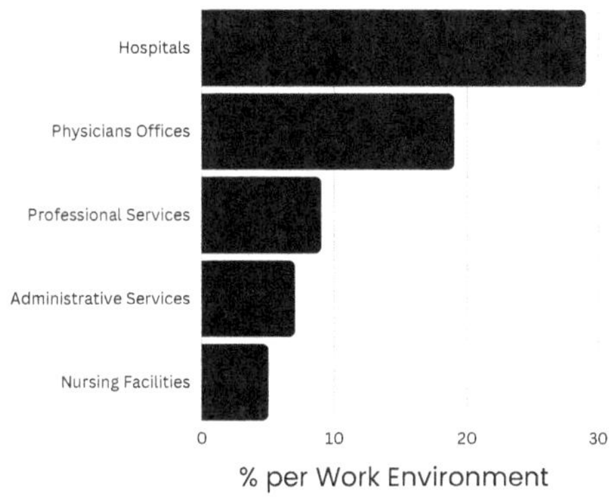

Resources:

- American Health Information Management Association: https://www.ahima.org/

Source: U.S. BUREAU OF LABOR STATISTICS

MEDICAL SCIENTISTS

OVERVIEW

Medical scientists conduct research aimed at improving overall human health. They often use clinical trials and other investigative methods to reach their findings.

Medical scientists form hypotheses and develop experiments. They study the causes of diseases and other health problems in a variety of ways and analyze data from clinical trials to evaluate results.

Some medical scientists choose to write about and publish their findings in scientific journals after completion of the clinical trial. They also may have to present their findings in ways that nonscientist audiences understand.

Medical scientists typically do the following:

- Design and conduct studies to investigate human diseases and methods to prevent and treat diseases
- Prepare and analyze data from medical samples and investigate causes and treatment of toxicity, pathogens, or chronic diseases
- Standardize drugs' potency, doses, and methods of administering to allow for their mass manufacturing and distribution
- Create and test medical devices
- Write articles for publication and present research findings

Education Level

Doctorate Degree

Type of Area

Non-Clinical

License or Certification

- None

Average Salary: $95k	Number of Jobs in 2021: 119,200
Average Hourly: $45/hr	Job Outlook in 2021: 17%
Salary Range: $50k to $166k	10y Change 2021 - 2031: 20,800

Education Requirements

- Bachelor's Degree (4 years)
- Doctorate of Philosophy (PhD)
- Doctorate of Medicine (MD), optional

Work Environment

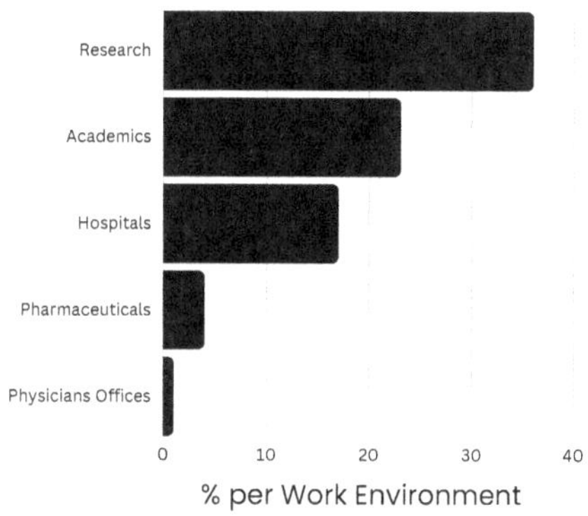

Resources:

- American Physician Scientists Association: https://www.physicianscientists.org/

Source: U.S. BUREAU OF LABOR STATISTICS

MEDICAL TRANSCRIPTIONISTS

OVERVIEW

Medical transcriptionists, sometimes referred to as healthcare documentation specialists, use electronic devices to convert voice recordings from physicians and other healthcare workers into formal reports. Transcriptionists also may edit medical records for accuracy and return documents for review and approval.

Medical transcriptionists use a variety of equipment to produce reports. The most common is speech recognition technology, which involves specialized software that automatically prepares an initial draft of a report that the transcriptionist reviews for accuracy.

Medical transcriptionists must be familiar with medical terminology, anatomy, and physiology. Transcriptionists' responsibilities are critical to preventing ineffective or harmful treatment.

Medical transcriptionists typically do the following:

- Listen to the recorded dictation of a physician or other healthcare worker
- Interpret and transcribe the dictation for medical reports, such as patient histories, discharge summaries, and physical examinations
- Review and edit drafts prepared by speech recognition software, making sure that the transcription is accurate, complete, and consistent in style
- Translate medical abbreviations and jargon into the appropriate long form
- Identify inconsistencies, errors, and missing information in a report that could compromise patient care

Education Level

Postsecondary Non-Degree

Type of Area

Non-Clinical

License or Certification

- None

Average Salary: **$30k**	**Number of Jobs in 2021:** **59,600**
Average Hourly: **$14/hr**	**Job Outlook in 2021:** **-7%**
Salary Range: **$22k to $48k**	**10y Change 2021 - 2031:** **-3,900**

Education Requirements

- Education Program (<1 year)

Work Environment

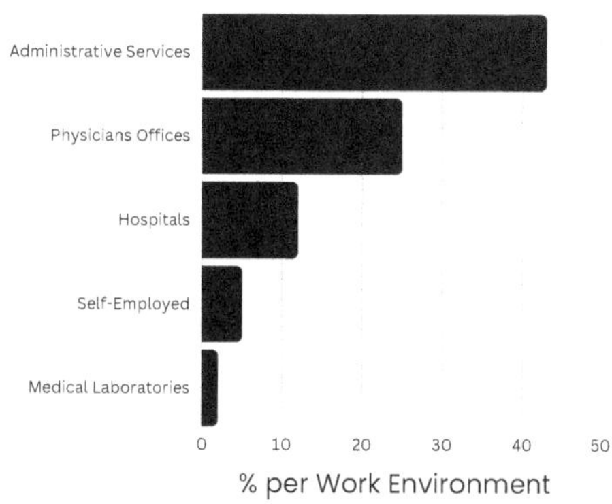

Resources:

- Association of Healthcare Documentation Integrity: https://www.ahdionline.org/

Source: U.S. BUREAU OF LABOR STATISTICS

MRI TECHNOLOGISTS

OVERVIEW

MRI technologists operate magnetic resonance imaging (MRI) scanners to create diagnostic images. MRI technologists specialize in magnetic resonance imaging scanners.

They inject patients with contrast media, such as a dye, so that the images will show up on the scanner. The scanners use magnetic fields in combination with the contrast agent to produce images that a physician can use to diagnose medical problems.

MRI Technologists typically do the following:

- Adjust and maintain imaging equipment
- Follow precise orders from physicians on what areas of the body to image
- Prepare patients for procedures, including taking a medical history and shielding exposed areas that do not need to be imaged
- Position the patient and the equipment in order to get the correct image
- Operate the computerized equipment to take the images
- Work with physicians to evaluate the images and to determine whether additional images need to be taken

Education Level

Associate's Degree

Type of Area

Clinical

License or Certification

- Depends on State

Average Salary: $77k	Number of Jobs in 2021: 41,200
Average Hourly: $37/hr	Job Outlook in 2021: 7%
Salary Range: $59k to $100k	10y Change 2021 - 2031: 3,000

Education Requirements

- Associate's Degree (2 years)

Work Environment

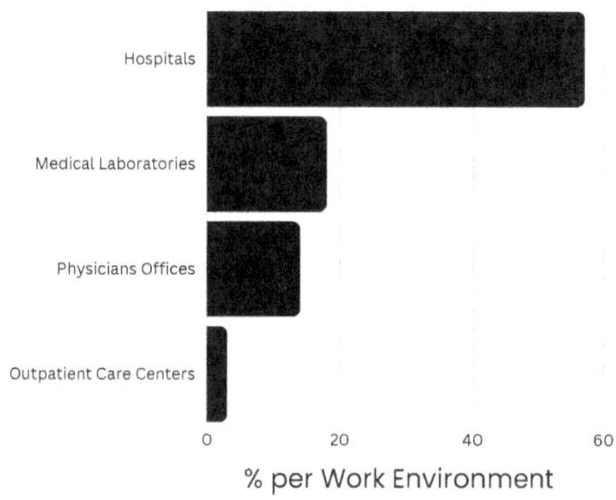

Resources:
- American Registry of Radiologic Technologists: https://www.arrt.org/
- American Society of Radiologic Technologists: https://www.asrt.org/

Source: U.S. BUREAU OF LABOR STATISTICS

MUSIC THERAPISTS

OVERVIEW

Music therapists use music interventions to help influence people and meet their goals. Through diverse music techniques music therapists help people reflect on and process various thoughts and feelings.

Music therapists work with a variety of children and adults that includes those with developmental disabilities, medical illnesses, physical disabilities, psychiatric disorders, or neurological impairments.

Music therapists typically do the following:

- Talk with clients about their symptoms, medical history, and treatment goals
- Evaluate clients prior to and during the music therapy
- Discuss music interventions with clients
- Help client's implement creative skills and techniques
- Provide guidance on self reflection and processing thoughts and feelings
- Document clients' conditions and progress

Education Level

Bachelor's Degree

Type of Area

Clinical

License or Certification

- Depends on State

Average Salary: **$71k***	**Number of Jobs in 2022:** **16,920***
Average Hourly: **$34/hr***	**Job Outlook in 2021:** **N/A**
Salary Range: **$37k to $111k***	**10y Change 2021 - 2031:** **N/A**

Education Requirements

- Bachelor's Degree (4 years)

Work Environment*

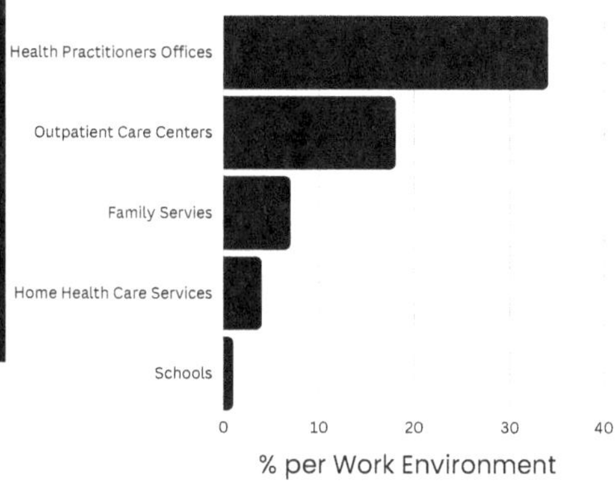

*Data from Therapists, All Other

Resources:

- American Music Therapy Association: https://www.musictherapy.org/about/musictherapy/

Source: U.S. BUREAU OF LABOR STATISTICS

NUCLEAR MEDICINE TECHNOLOGISTS

OVERVIEW

Nuclear medicine technologists prepare radioactive drugs and administer them to patients for imaging or treatment. They provide technical support to physicians or others who diagnose, care for, and treat patients and to researchers who investigate uses of radioactive drugs. They also may act as emergency responders in the event of a nuclear disaster.

Nuclear medicine technologists work with radioactive drugs, known as radiopharmaceuticals, to help physicians and surgeons diagnose a patient's condition. They inject radiopharmaceuticals into the bloodstream of the area of focus then use special scanning equipment that captures images.

Nuclear medicine technologists also deliver radiopharmaceuticals in prescribed doses to specific areas, such as tumors, to treat medical conditions. Internal radiation treatment may be used in conjunction with, or as an alternative to, surgery.

Nuclear medicine technologists typically do the following:

- Explain medical procedures to the patient and answer questions
- Follow safety procedures to protect themselves and the patient from unnecessary radiation exposure
- Prepare radioactive drugs and administer them to the patient
- Maintain and operate imaging equipment
- Keep detailed records of procedures
- Follow procedures for radiation disposal

Education Level

Associate's Degree

Type of Area

Clinical

License or Certification

- Depends on State

Average Salary: $78k
Average Hourly: $37/hr
Salary Range: $60k to $105k

Number of Jobs in 2021: 18,900
Job Outlook in 2021: 2%
10y Change 2021 - 2031: 300

Education Requirements

- Associate's Degree (2 years)

Work Environment

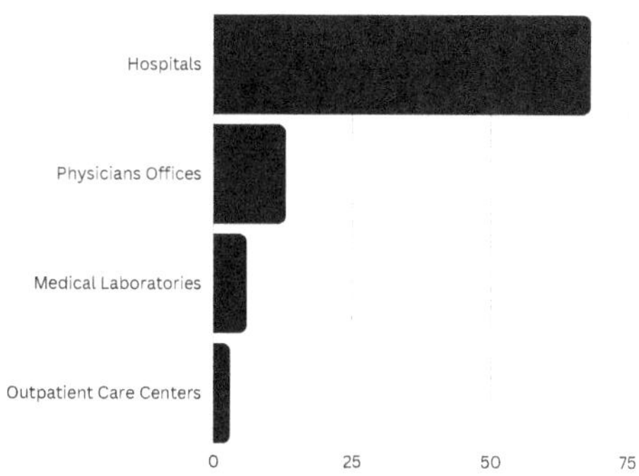

Note: Types of nuclear medicine technologists include Nuclear cardiology technologists, Nuclear medicine computed tomography (CT) technologists, and Positron emission tomography (PET) technologists.

Resources:

- American Society of Radiologic Technologists: https://www.asrt.org/
- Society of Nuclear Medicine and Molecular Imaging: https://www.snmmi.org/

Source: U.S. BUREAU OF LABOR STATISTICS

NURSE ANESTHETISTS

OVERVIEW

Nurse anesthetists, nurse midwives, and nurse practitioners, also referred to as advanced practice registered nurses (APRNs), coordinate patient care and may provide primary and specialty healthcare.

Nurse anesthetists (CRNAs) administer anesthesia and provide care before, during, and after surgical, therapeutic, diagnostic, and obstetrical procedures. They also provide pain management and some emergency services.

Nurse anesthetists give patients general anesthesia to put the patient to sleep so they feel no pain during surgery or administer a regional or local anesthesia to numb an area of the body. During the procedure, they monitor the patient's vital signs and adjust the anesthesia as necessary.

Advanced practice registered nurses typically do the following:

- Take and record patients' medical histories and symptoms
- Perform physical exams and observe patients
- Perform and order diagnostic tests
- Operate and monitor medical equipment
- Diagnose various health problems
- Analyze test results or changes in a patient's condition and alter treatment plans, as needed
- Give and evaluate a patient's response to medicines and treatments
- Consult with doctors and other healthcare professionals, as needed
- Counsel and teach patients and their families how to stay healthy or manage their illnesses or injuries

Education Level

Master's Degree

Type of Area

Clinical

License or Certification

- State License

Average Salary: $203k	**Number of Jobs in 2021:** 45,200
Average Hourly: $97/hr	**Job Outlook in 2021:** 12%
Salary Range:* $91k to $208k	**10y Change 2021 - 2031:** 5,300

Education Requirements

- Associate's Degree (2 years) or Bachelor's Degree (4 years)
- Master's Degree (2-4 years)

Work Environment

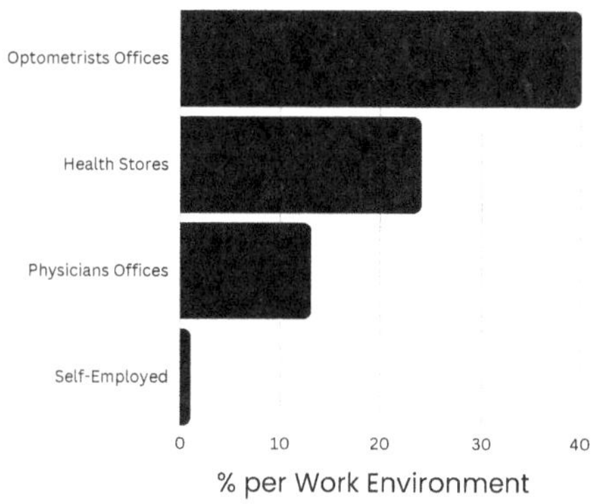

*Salary range for Nurse Anesthetists, Nurse Midwives, and Nurse Practitioners

Resources

- American Association of Nurse Anesthetists: https://www.aana.com/

Source: U.S. BUREAU OF LABOR STATISTICS

NURSING ASSISTANTS

OVERVIEW

Nursing assistants, sometimes called nursing aides, provide basic care and help patients with activities of daily living. Depending on their training level and the state in which they work, nursing assistants also may dispense medication.

Nursing assistants are often the principal caregivers in nursing and residential care facilities. Nursing assistants often develop relationships with their patients because some patients stay in these facilities for months or years.

Nursing assistants typically do the following:

- Clean and bathe patients
- Help patients use the toilet and dress
- Turn, reposition, and transfer patients between beds and wheelchairs
- Listen to and record patients' health concerns and report that information to nurses
- Measure patients' vital signs, such as blood pressure and temperature
- Serve meals and help patients eat

Education Level

Postsecondary Non-Degree

Type of Area

Clinical

License or Certification

- State License

Average Salary: $30k	Number of Jobs in 2021: 1,389,900
Average Hourly: $14/hr	Job Outlook in 2021: 5%
Salary Range: $23k to $44k	10y Change 2021 - 2031: 64,900

Education Requirements

- Education Program (4-12 weeks)

Work Environment

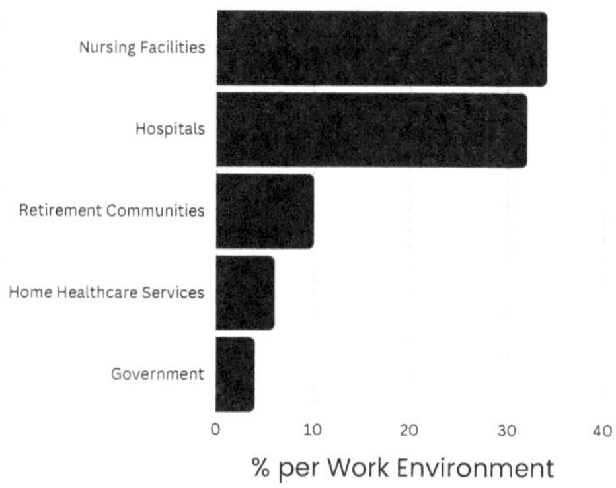

Note: Orderlies typically do the following: Help patients to move around the facility, such as by pushing their wheelchairs; Clean equipment and facilities; Change linens; and Stock supplies. Orderlies typically have at least a high school diploma or equivalent.

Resources:

- National Association of Health Care Assistants: https://www.nahcacna.org/

Source: U.S. BUREAU OF LABOR STATISTICS

NURSE MIDWIVES

OVERVIEW

Nurse anesthetists, nurse midwives, and nurse practitioners, also referred to as advanced practice registered nurses (APRNs), coordinate patient care and may provide primary and specialty healthcare.

Nurse midwives (CNMs) provide care to women, including gynecological exams, family planning services, and prenatal care. They deliver babies, manage emergency situations during labor, repair lacerations, and may provide surgical assistance to physicians during cesarean births.

Nurse midwives may act as primary maternity care providers for women. They also provide wellness care, educating their patients on how to lead healthy lives by discussing topics such as nutrition and disease prevention.

Advanced practice registered nurses typically do the following:

- Take and record patients' medical histories and symptoms
- Perform physical exams and observe patients
- Create patient care plans or contribute to existing plans
- Perform and order diagnostic tests
- Diagnose various health problems
- Analyze test results or changes in a patient's condition and alter treatment plans, as needed
- Give and evaluate a patient's response to medicines and treatments
- Consult with doctors and other healthcare professionals, as needed
- Counsel and teach patients and their families how to stay healthy or manage their illnesses or injuries

Education Level

Master's Degree

Type of Area

Clinical

License or Certification

- State License

Average Salary: $120k	Number of Jobs in 2021: 8,100
Average Hourly: $57/hr	Job Outlook in 2021: 7%
Salary Range:* $91k to $208k	10y Change 2021 - 2031: 600

Education Requirements

- Associate's Degree (2 years) or Bachelor's Degree (4 years)
- Master's Degree (2-4 years)

Work Environment

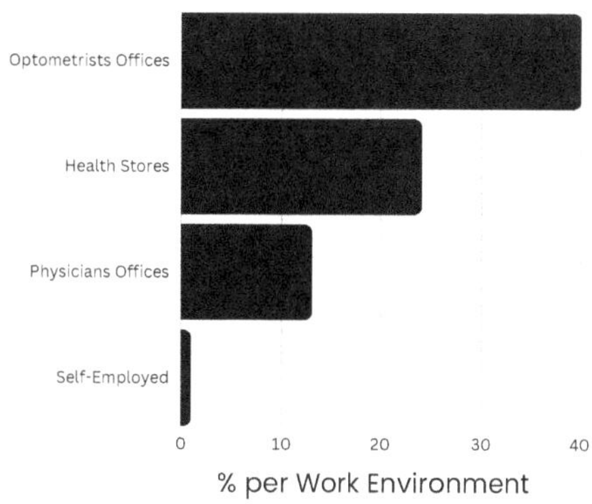

*Salary range for Nurse Anesthetists, Nurse Midwives, and Nurse Practitioners

Resources:

- American College of Nurse-Midwives: http://www.midwife.org/
- National Association of Certified Professional Midwives: https://www.nacpm.org/

Source: U.S. BUREAU OF LABOR STATISTICS

NURSE PRACTITIONERS

OVERVIEW

Nurse anesthetists, nurse midwives, and nurse practitioners, also referred to as advanced practice registered nurses (APRNs), coordinate patient care and may provide primary and specialty healthcare.

Nurse practitioners (NPs) serve as primary and specialty care providers, delivering advanced nursing services to patients and their families. They assess patients, determine how to improve or manage a patient's health, and discuss ways to integrate health promotion strategies into a patient's life. Nurse practitioners typically care for a certain population of people such as pediatric health, adult health, or psychiatric health.

Advanced practice registered nurses typically do the following:

- Take and record patients' medical histories and symptoms
- Perform physical exams and observe patients
- Create patient care plans or contribute to existing plans
- Perform and order diagnostic tests
- Operate and monitor medical equipment
- Diagnose various health problems
- Analyze test results or changes in a patient's condition and alter treatment plans, as needed
- Give and evaluate a patient's response to medicines and treatments
- Consult with doctors and other healthcare professionals, as needed
- Counsel and teach patients and their families how to stay healthy or manage their illnesses or injuries

Education Level

Master's Degree

Type of Area

Clinical

License or Certification

- State License

Average Salary: $121k
Average Hourly: $58/hr
Salary Range:* $91k to $208k

Number of Jobs in 2021: 246,700
Job Outlook in 2021: 46%
10y Change 2021 - 2031: 112,700

Education Requirements

- Associate's Degree (2 years) or Bachelor's Degree (4 years)
- Master's Degree (2-4 years)

Work Environment

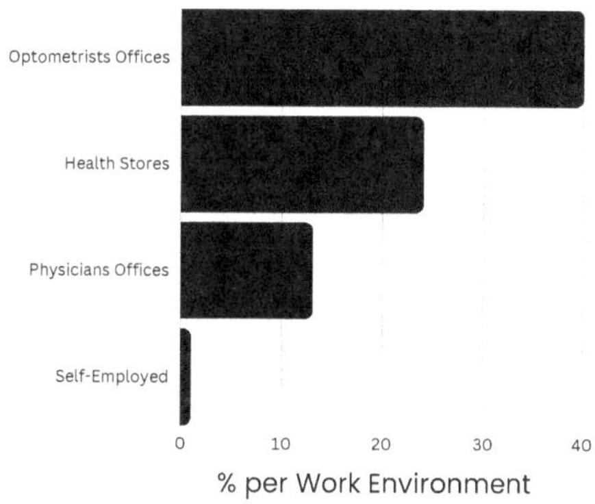

*Salary range for Nurse Anesthetists, Nurse Midwives, and Nurse Practitioners

Resources:

- American Association of Nurse Practitioners: https://www.aanp.org/

Source: U.S. BUREAU OF LABOR STATISTICS

OCCUPATIONAL THERAPISTS

OVERVIEW

Occupational therapists evaluate and treat people who have injuries, illnesses, or disabilities. They help clients meet goals to develop, recover, improve, and maintain skills needed for daily living and working.

Occupational therapists work with people who have permanent disabilities and may need help with daily tasks. They recommend options and show clients how to use appropriate adaptive equipment that help clients live their lives more independently.

Occupational therapists typically do the following:

- Evaluate clients' conditions by reviewing their medical history, interviewing them, and observing them perform various tasks
- Develop and implement treatment plans that have specific activities to help clients work toward their goals
- Help clients relearn and perform daily living tasks
- Evaluate a client's home, school, or workplace to identify potential accessibility improvements
- Educate a client's family about how to accommodate and care for them
- Recommend special equipment and instruct clients on how to use it

Education Level

Master's Degree

Type of Area

Clinical

License or Certification

- State License
- National Board for Certification in Occupatio[nal] Therapy (NBCOT) Exam

Average Salary: $85k	Number of Jobs in 2021: 133,900
Average Hourly: $41/hr	Job Outlook in 2021: 14%
Salary Range: $60k to $123k	10y Change 2021 - 2031: 18,600

Education Requirements

- Bachelor's Degree (4 years)
- Master's Degree (2-3 years)

Work Environment

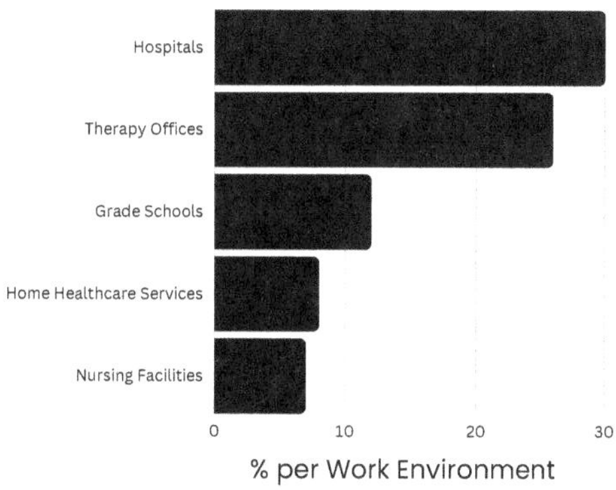

Resources:

- American Occupational Therapists Association: https://www.aotf.org/

Source: U.S. BUREAU OF LABOR STATISTICS

OCCUPATIONAL THERAPIST ASSISTANTS

OVERVIEW

Occupational therapy assistants and aides help patients develop, recover, improve, as well as maintain the skills needed for daily living and working. Occupational therapy assistants are directly involved in providing therapy to patients while working under the direction of occupational therapists.

Occupational therapy assistants collaborate with occupational therapists to develop and carry out a treatment plan for each patient. Plans include diverse activities such as teaching the proper ways to adapt to injured or lost motor skills. Occupational therapy assistants also may work with people who have learning disabilities, teaching them skills that allow them to be more independent.

Occupational therapy assistants typically do the following:

- Help patients do therapeutic activities, such as stretches and other exercises
- Lead children who have developmental disabilities in play activities that promote coordination and socialization
- Encourage patients to complete activities and tasks
- Teach patients how to use special equipment to assist in movements
- Record patients' progress, report to occupational therapists, and do other administrative tasks

Education Level

Associate's Degree

Type of Area

Clinical

License or Certification

- State License

Average Salary: $61k
Average Hourly: $29/hr
Salary Range: $46k to $80k

Number of Jobs in 2021: 47,000
Job Outlook in 2021: 25%
10y Change 2021 - 2031: 11,500

Work Environment

Education Requirements

- Associate's Degree (2 years)

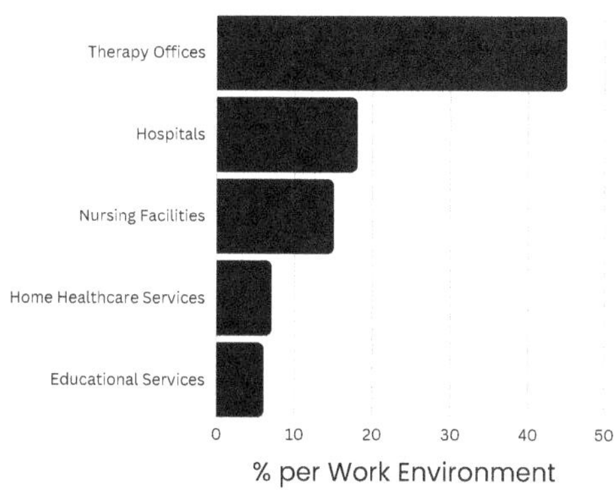

Note: Occupational therapy aides typically prepare materials and assemble equipment used during treatment. They may assist patients with moving to and from treatment areas. They fill out insurance forms and other paperwork and are responsible for a range of clerical tasks. Occupational therapy aides typically need a high school diploma or equivalent and are trained on the job.

Resources:

- American Occupational Therapists Association: https://www.aotf.org/

Source: U.S. BUREAU OF LABOR STATISTICS

OPTICIANS

OVERVIEW

Opticians help fit eyeglasses and contact lenses, following prescriptions from ophthalmologists and optometrists. They also help customers decide which eyeglass frames or contact lenses to buy.

Opticians typically do the following:

- Receive customers' prescriptions for eyeglasses or contact lenses
- Measure customers' eyes and faces, such as the distance between their pupils
- Help customers choose eyeglass frames and lens treatments
- Create work orders for ophthalmic laboratory technicians, providing information about the lenses needed
- Adjust eyewear to ensure a good fit
- Repair or replace broken eyeglass frames
- Educate customers about eyewear
- Perform business tasks, such as maintaining sales records, keeping track of customers' prescriptions, and ordering and maintaining inventory

Education Level

High School Diploma

Type of Area

Clinical

License or Certification

- Depends on State

Average Salary: $37k	Number of Jobs in 2021: 74,800
Average Hourly: $18/hr	Job Outlook in 2021: 4%
Salary Range: $28k to $60k	10y Change 2021 - 2031: 2,800

Education Requirements

- On the Job Training or Associate's Degree (2 years)

Work Environment

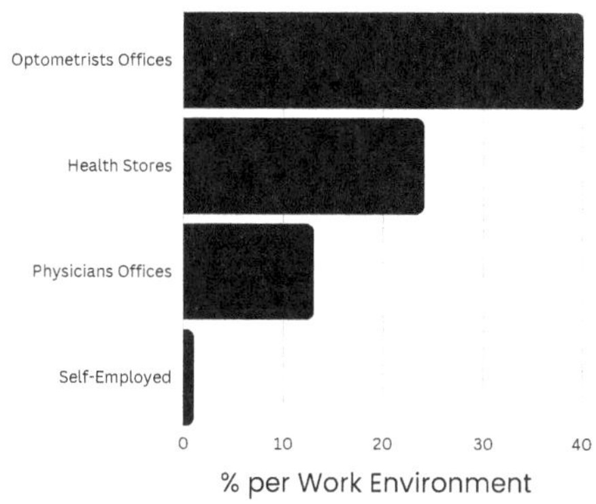

Resources:

- Opticians Association of America: https://oaa.org/

Source: U.S. BUREAU OF LABOR STATISTICS

OPTOMETRISTS

OVERVIEW

Optometrists diagnose, manage, and treat conditions and diseases of the human eye and visual system, including examining eyes and prescribing corrective lenses.

Optometrists are doctors who focus on eyes and vision. Their tasks range from offering preventive care through routine checkups to providing referrals to other specialists for treatment of health conditions that may lead to serious eye problems.

Some optometrists provide specialized care in addition to general eye care. Others may specialize in treating a certain population, such as infants and children.

Optometrists typically do the following:

- Perform vision tests and analyze results
- Diagnose vision problems, such as nearsightedness or farsightedness, and eye diseases, such as glaucoma
- Prescribe eyeglasses, contact lenses, and other visual aids
- As permitted by state law, perform minor surgical procedures and prescribe medications to correct or treat visual or eye issues
- Provide treatments such as vision therapy or low-vision rehabilitation
- Provide pre- and postoperative care to patients undergoing eye surgery
- Evaluate patients for the presence of other diseases and conditions and refer patients to other healthcare providers as needed
- Promote eye and general health by counseling patients

Education Level

Doctorate Degree

Type of Area

Clinical

License or Certification

- State License
- National Board of Examine in Optometry Exam

Average Salary: $124k	Number of Jobs in 2021: 41,400
Average Hourly: $59/hr	Job Outlook in 2021: 10%
Salary Range: $61k to $192k	10y Change 2021 - 2031: 4,000

Education Requirements

- Bachelor's Degree (4 years)
- Doctor of Optometry (4 years, O.D)

Work Environment

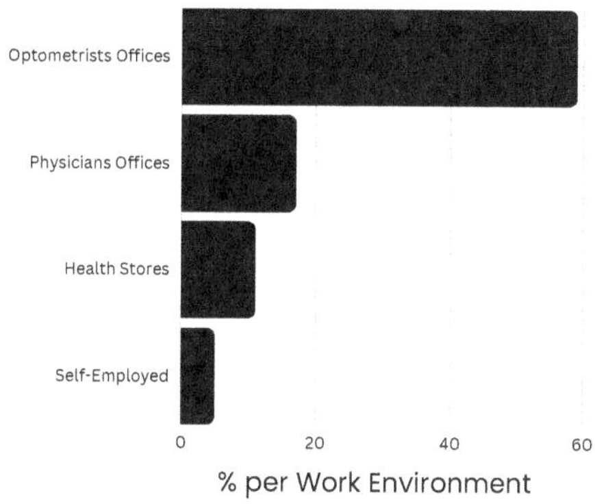

Note: Optometrists should not be confused with ophthalmologists or opticians. Ophthalmologists are physicians who, like optometrists, treat eye diseases, perform eye exams, and prescribe eyeglasses and contact lenses. However, ophthalmologists perform a wider range of surgeries than optometrists do.

Resources:

- American Academy of Optometry: https://aaopt.org/
- American Optometric Association: https://www.aoa.org/

Source: U.S. BUREAU OF LABOR STATISTICS

ORTHOTISTS AND PROSTHETISTS

OVERVIEW

Orthotists and prosthetists design and fabricate medical supportive devices and measure and fit patients for them. These devices include artificial limbs (arms, hands, legs, and feet), braces, and other medical or surgical devices.

Orthotists and prosthetists may work in both orthotics and prosthetics, or they may choose to specialize in one area. Orthotists are specifically trained to work with medical supportive devices, such as spinal or knee braces. Prosthetists are specifically trained to work with prostheses, such as artificial limbs and other body parts.

Some orthotists and prosthetists construct devices for their patients. Others supervise the construction of the orthotic or prosthetic devices by medical appliance technicians.

Orthotists and Prosthetists typically do the following:

- Evaluate and interview patients to determine their needs
- Take measurements or impressions of the part of a patient's body that will be fitted with a brace or artificial limb
- Design and fabricate orthopedic and prosthetic devices based on physicians' prescriptions
- Select materials to be used for the orthotic or prosthetic device
- Instruct patients in how to use and care for their devices
- Adjust, repair, or replace prosthetic and orthotic devices

Education Level

Master's Degree

Type of Area

Clinical

License or Certification

- Depends on State

Average Salary: $75k	Number of Jobs in 2021: 11,100
Average Hourly: $36/hr	Job Outlook in 2021: 17%
Salary Range: $41k to $124k	10y Change 2021 - 2031: 1,900

Education Requirements

- Bachelor's Degree (4 years)
- Master's Degree (2 years)
- Residency Training (1 year)

Work Environment

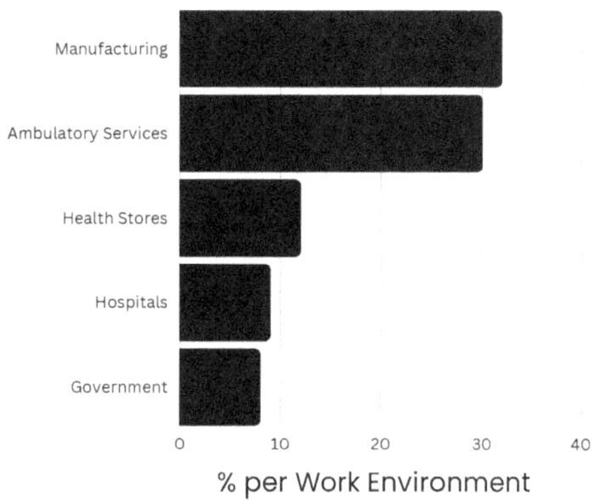

Resources:

- American Orthotic and Prosthetic Association: https://www.aopanet.org/
- American Academy of Orthotists and Prosthetists: https://www.oandp.org/

Source: U.S. BUREAU OF LABOR STATISTICS

PHARMACISTS

OVERVIEW

Pharmacists dispense prescription medications and provide information to patients about the drugs and their use. They also advise physicians and other healthcare workers on the selection, dosage, interactions, and side effects of medications to treat health problems.

They may help patients with their overall health through activities such as providing immunizations. Pharmacists may answer patients' questions about their prescriptions and the use of over-the-counter medications.

Pharmacists verify instructions from physicians to fill and dispense prescription medications. They also may create customized medications by mixing ingredients themselves, a process known as compounding.

Pharmacists typically do the following:

- Fill prescriptions to the proper amount based on physicians' instructions
- Check patients' allergies, medical conditions, and other drugs they are taking to ensure that the newly prescribed medication does not cause adverse reaction
- Instruct patients on proper use, side effects, and storage of prescribed medicine
- Administer vaccinations
- Advise patients about general health topics and on other issues, such as what equipment or supplies would be best to treat a health problem
- Maintain patient and pharmacy records
- Educate other healthcare workers about proper medication therapies for patients

Education Level

Doctorate Degree

Type of Area

Clinical

License or Certification

- State License
- North American Pharmaci
Licensing Exam (NAPLEX)
- Multi-State Pharmacy
Jurisprudence Exam (MPJ

Average Salary: $128k	Number of Jobs in 2021: 323,500
Average Hourly: $61/hr	Job Outlook in 2021: 2%
Salary Range: $76k to $164k	10y Change 2021 - 2031: 7,700

Education Requirements

- Bachelor's Degree (4 years)
- Doctor of Pharmacy (4 years, PharmD)
- Post-Doctoral Training (1-2 years), optional

Work Environment

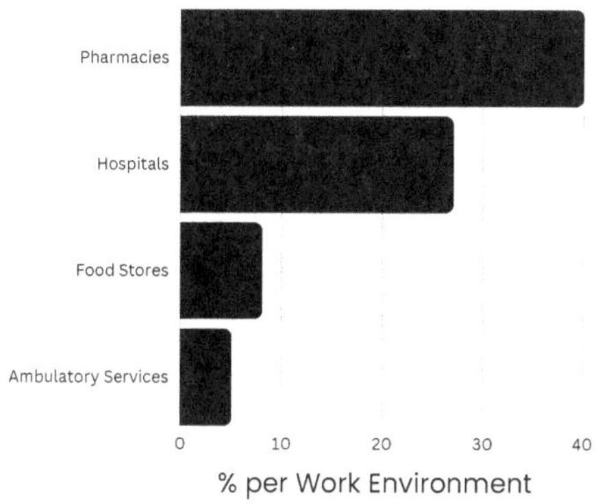

Note: Types of pharmacists includes Community pharmacists, Clinical pharmacists, Consultant pharmacists, and Pharmaceutical industry pharmacists.

Resources:

- American Pharmacists Association: https://www.pharmacist.com/

Source: U.S. BUREAU OF LABOR STATISTICS

PHARMACY TECHNICIANS

OVERVIEW

Pharmacy technicians help pharmacists dispense prescription medication to customers or health professionals. They mainly work in retail pharmacies and hospitals.

Pharmacy technicians work under the supervision of pharmacists, who must review prescriptions before they are given to patients. In most states, technicians can compound or mix some medications and call physicians for prescription refill authorizations.

Pharmacy technicians working in hospitals and other medical facilities prepare a greater variety of medications, such as intravenous medications. They may make rounds in the hospital, giving medications to patients.

Pharmacy technicians typically do the following:

- Collect information needed to fill a prescription from customers or health professionals
- Measure amounts of medication for prescriptions
- Package and label prescriptions
- Organize inventory and alert pharmacists to any shortages of medications or supplies
- Accept payment for prescriptions and process insurance claims
- Answer phone calls from customers
- Arrange for customers to speak with pharmacists if customers have questions about medications or health matters

Education Level

High School Diploma

Type of Area

Clinical

License or Certification

- Depends on State

Average Salary: $36k	**Number of Jobs in 2021:** 447,300
Average Hourly: $17/hr	**Job Outlook in 2021:** 5%
Salary Range: $28k to $47k	**10y Change 2021 - 2031:** 22,400

Education Requirements

- On the Job Training or Education Program (1 year)

Work Environment

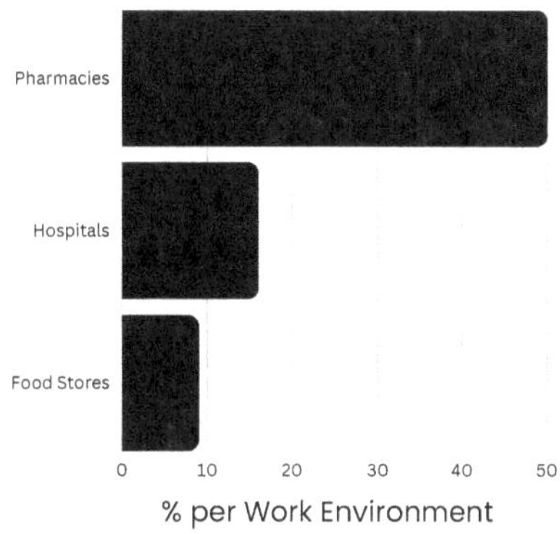

Resources:

- National Pharmacy Technician Association: http://www.pharmacytechnician.org/
- American Association of Pharmacy Technicians: http://www.pharmacytechnician.com/

Source: U.S. BUREAU OF LABOR STATISTICS

PHLEBOTOMISTS

OVERVIEW

Phlebotomists draw blood for purposes such as tests, research, or donations. They help patients or donors who are anxious before or have an adverse reaction after the blood draw.

Phlebotomists primarily draw blood, which is then used for different kinds of medical laboratory testing or for procedures, such as transfusions. Because all blood looks the same, phlebotomists must carefully identify and label the blood they have collected and enter the information into a database.

In addition to drawing blood, phlebotomists also may collect urine or other samples. They instruct patients on procedures for proper collection and ensure that the sample is acceptable and clearly labeled in its container.

Phlebotomists typically do the following:

- Draw blood from patients or blood donors
- Explain their work to help relax patients or donors who feel nervous about having blood drawn
- Verify a patient's or donor's identity
- Label the collected blood for testing or processing
- Label sterile containers for other samples, such as urine, and instruct patients on proper collection procedures.
- Enter sample information into a database
- Assemble, maintain, and dispose of medical instruments such as needles, test tubes, and blood vials

Education Level

Post Secondary Non-Degree

Type of Area

Clinical

License or Certification

- Depends on State and Employment

Average Salary: $37k	Number of Jobs in 2021: 135,500
Average Hourly: $18/hr	Job Outlook in 2021: 10%
Salary Range: $28k to $48k	10y Change 2021 - 2031: 13,900

Education Requirements

- Education Program (1 year)

Work Environment

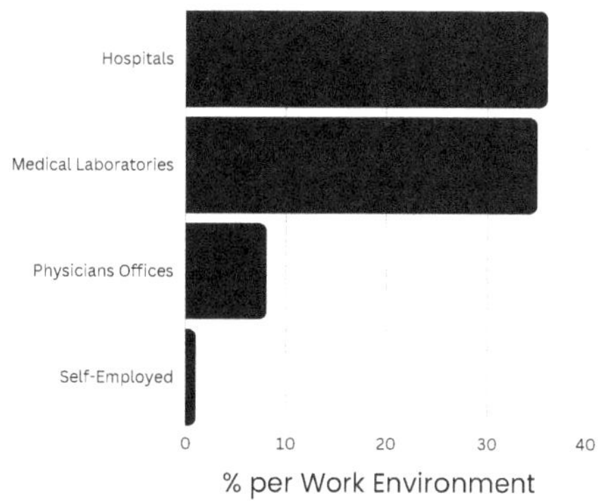

Resources:

- National Phlebotomy Association: https://www.nationalphlebotomy.org/
- American Society of Phlebotomy Technicians: https://www.aspt.org/

Source: U.S. BUREAU OF LABOR STATISTICS

PHYSICAL THERAPISTS

OVERVIEW

Physical therapists help injured or ill people improve movement and manage pain. They are often an important part of preventive care, rehabilitation, and treatment for patients with chronic conditions, illnesses, or injuries.

Physical therapists, sometimes called PTs, care for people of all ages who have functional problems resulting conditions like back and neck injuries, sprains, fractures, arthritis, amputations, and neurological disorders. Physical therapists use a variety of techniques and equipment to care for their patients.

Physical therapists typically do the following:

- Review patients' medical history and referrals or notes from doctors, surgeons, or other healthcare workers
- Diagnose patients' functions and movements by observing them stand or walk and by listening to their concerns
- Develop plans of care for patients, outlining the patients' goals and the expected outcomes of the plans
- Use exercises, stretching maneuvers, hands-on therapy, and equipment to ease patients' pain, help them increase their mobility, prevent further pain or injury, and facilitate health and wellness
- Evaluate and record a patients' progress, modifying the plan of care and trying new treatments as needed
- Educate patients and their families

Education Level

Doctorate Degree

Type of Area

Clinical

License or Certification

- State License
- National Physical Therapy Examination

Average Salary: $95k	Number of Jobs in 2021: 238,800
Average Hourly: $45/hr	Job Outlook in 2021: 17%
Salary Range: $61k to $127k	10y Change 2021 - 2031: 40,400

Education Requirements

- Bachelor's Degree (4 years)
- Doctor of Physical Therapy (3 years, DPT)

Work Environment

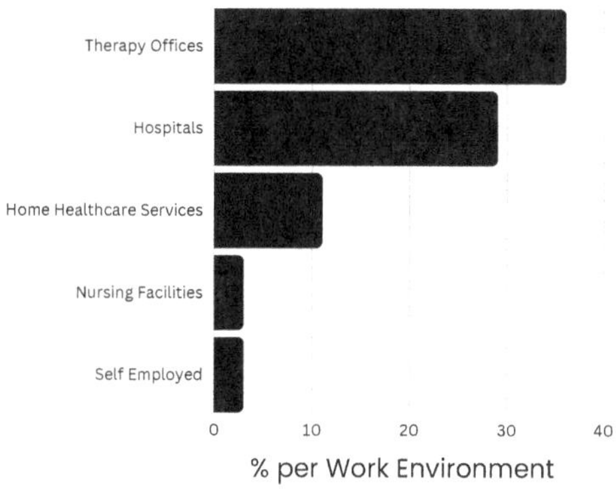

Resources:

- American Physical Therapy Association: https://www.apta.org/

Source: U.S. BUREAU OF LABOR STATISTICS

PHYSICAL THERAPIST ASSISTANTS

OVERVIEW

Physical therapist assistants, sometimes called PTAs, and physical therapist aides work under the direction and supervision of physical therapists. They help patients who are recovering from injuries and illnesses to regain movement and manage pain.

Physical therapist assistants treat patients through exercise, massage, gait and balance training, and other therapeutic interventions. They record patients' progress and report the results of each treatment to the physical therapist.

Physical therapists assistants typically do the following:

- Observe patients before, during, and after therapy, noting the patient's status and reporting it to a physical therapist
- Help patients do specific exercises as part of the plan of care
- Treat patients using a variety of techniques, such as massage and stretching
- Use devices and equipment, such as walkers, to help patients
- Educate patients and family members about what to do after treatment
- Under the direction and supervision of physical therapists, physical therapist assistants treat patients through exercise, massage, gait and balance training, and other therapeutic interventions.

Education Level

Associate's Degree

Type of Area

Clinical

License or Certification

- State License
- National Physical Therapy Exam for PTAs

Average Salary: **$61k**	**Number of Jobs in 2021:** **140,800**
Average Hourly: **$29/hr**	**Job Outlook in 2021:** **24%**
Salary Range: **$37k to $80k**	**10y Change 2021 - 2031:** **33,900**

Education Requirements

- Associate's Degree (2 years)

Work Environment

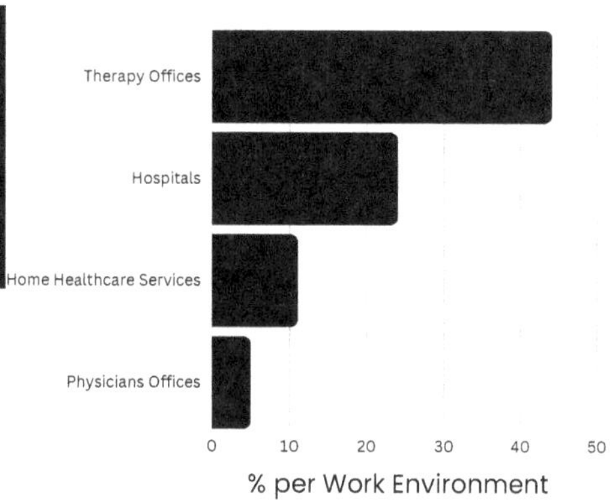

Note: Physical therapist aides often have tasks that are indirectly related to patient care, such as cleaning and setting up the treatment area, moving patients, and doing clerical duties. Physical therapist aides usually need a high school diploma or equivalent and on-the-job training.

Resources:

- American Physical Therapy Association: https://www.apta.org/

Source: U.S. BUREAU OF LABOR STATISTICS

PHYSICIANS AND SURGEONS

OVERVIEW

Physicians and surgeons diagnose and treat injuries or illnesses and address health maintenance. Physicians examine patients; take medical histories; prescribe medications; and order, perform, and interpret diagnostic tests. Surgeons are physicians that operate on patients to treat injuries, diseases, and deformities.

There are two types of physicians, with similar degrees: M.D. (Medical Doctor) and D.O. (Doctor of Osteopathic Medicine). Both use the same methods of treatment, including drugs and surgery, but D.O.s place additional emphasis on the body's musculoskeletal system, preventive medicine, and holistic (whole-person) patient care.

Physicians and surgeons typically do the following:

- Take a patient's medical history and perform a physical exam
- Document and update charts and patient information to show findings and treatments
- Order tests and consultations for other physicians or healthcare staff to perform
- Review test results to identify abnormal findings
- Recommend, design, and implement a treatment plan
- Address concerns or answer questions that patients have about their health and well-being
- Help patients take care of their health by discussing topics such as proper nutrition and hygiene

Education Level

Doctorate Degree

Type of Area

Clinical

License or Certification

- State License
- U.S. Medical Licensing Examination (USMLE)
- Comprehensive Osteopathic Medical Licensing Examination (COMLEX-USA)

Average Salary: $208k	Number of Jobs in 2021: 761,700
Average Hourly: $100/hr	Job Outlook in 2021: 3%
Salary Range: $150k to $600k+	10y Change 2021 - 2031: 21,400

Education Requirements

- Bachelor's degree (4 years)
- Doctorate in Medicine degree (4 years) or Doctor of Osteopathic Medicine (4 years)
- Internship/Residency Program (3 to 9 years)
- Fellowship Training (1 to 3 years), if subspecialization

Work Environment

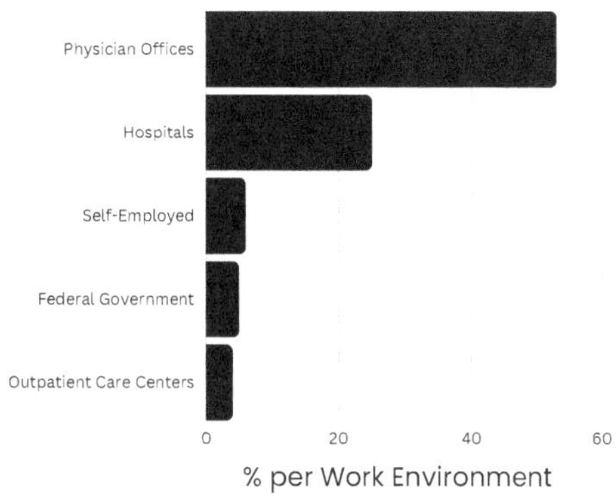

Note: There are over 15 specialities that physicians can pursue that are classified as medical, surgical, or both. During medical school students determine their desired speciality and pursue a Residency program for speciality training.

Resources:

- American Medical Association: https://www.ama-assn.org/

Source: U.S. BUREAU OF LABOR STATISTICS

PHYSICIAN ASSISTANTS

OVERVIEW

Physician assistants examine, diagnose, and treat patients under the supervision of a physician.

Physician assistants are on teams with physicians or surgeons and other healthcare workers. The amount of collaboration and the extent to which they must be supervised by physicians or surgeons differ by state.

Physician assistants work in a variety of healthcare specialties, including primary care and family medicine, emergency medicine, and psychiatry. The work of physician assistants depends, in large part, on their specialty or the type of medical practice in which they work.

Physician assistants typically do the following:

- Obtain and review patients' medical histories
- Examine patients
- Order and interpret diagnostic tests, such as x-rays or blood tests
- Diagnose a patient's injury or illness
- Provide treatment, such as setting broken bones, stitching wounds, and immunizing patients
- Educate and counsel patients and their families on a variety of issues, such as treatment and self-care for asthma
- Prescribe medication
- Assess and record a patient's progress
- Research the latest treatments to ensure quality of patient care

Education Level

Master's Degree

Type of Area

Clinical

License or Certification

- State License
- Physician Assistant National Certifying Examination (PANCE)

Average Salary: **$121k**
Average Hourly: **$58/hr**
Salary Range: **$77k to $164k**

Number of Jobs in 2021: **139,100**
Job Outlook in 2021: **28%**
10y Change 2021 - 2031: **38,400**

Education Requirements

- Bachelor's degree (4 years)
- Master's Degree (2 years)
- Postgraduate Program, optional

Work Environment

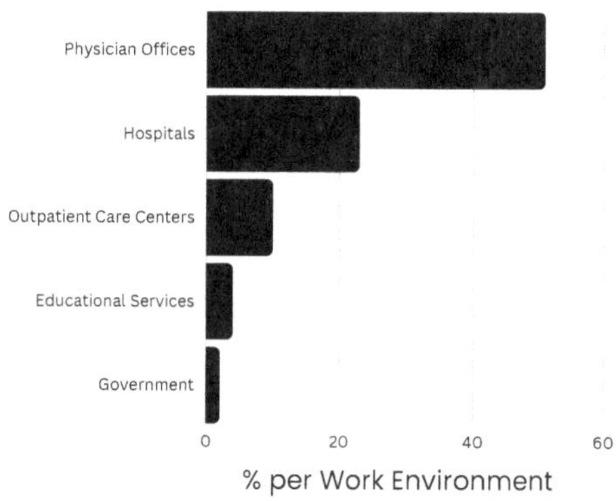

Note: Some physician assistants pursue additional education in a specialty. Postgraduate programs are available in specialties such as emergency medicine and psychiatry.

Resources:

- American Academy of Physician Assistants: https://www.aapa.org/

Source: U.S. BUREAU OF LABOR STATISTICS

PODIATRISTS

OVERVIEW

Podiatrists diagnose illnesses, treat injuries, and perform surgery for people with foot, ankle, and lower leg problems.

Podiatrists treat a variety of foot and ankle ailments, including calluses, ingrown toenails, heel spurs, arthritis, and arch problems. They also treat foot and leg problems associated with diabetes, obesity, and other health conditions.

Some podiatrists spend most of their time performing surgery, such as foot and ankle reconstruction. Others may choose a specialty such as sports medicine, pediatrics, or diabetic foot care.

Podiatrists typically do the following:

- Diagnose and assess patients' conditions by reviewing medical histories, performing physical exams, and reviewing x-rays and medical laboratory tests.
- Provide nonsurgical treatment for foot, ankle, and lower leg ailments, such as prescribing special shoe inserts (orthotics) to improve a patient's mobility
- Perform foot and ankle surgeries, such as removing bone spurs, repairing fractures, and correcting other foot and ankle problems
- Advise and instruct patients about foot and ankle care and wellness
- Prescribe medications
- Refer patients to other physicians or specialists if they detect other health problems, such as diabetes or vascular disease

Education Level

Doctorate Degree

Type of Area

Clinical

License or Certification

- State License
- American Podiatric Medical Licensing Exam (APMLE)

Average Salary: $145k	Number of Jobs in 2021: 11,000
Average Hourly: $70/hr	Job Outlook in 2021: 2%
Salary Range: $61k to $208k	10y Change 2021 - 2031: 200

Education Requirements

- Bachelor's Degree
- Doctor of Podiatric Medicine (4 years, DPM)
- Residency Training (3 years)

Work Environment

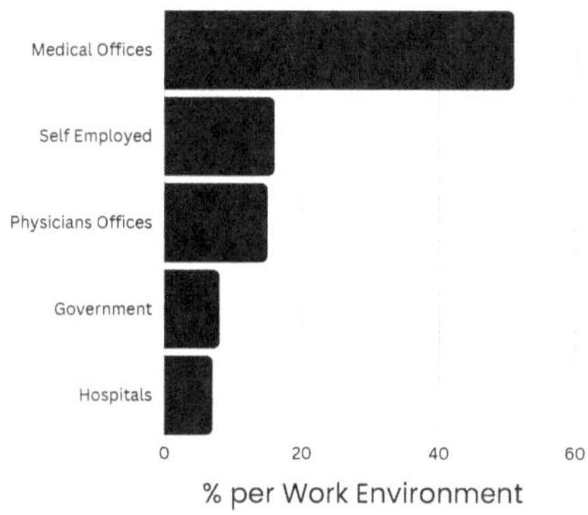

Resources:

- American Podiatric Medical Association: https://www.apma.org/
- American Society of Podiatric Surgeons: https://www.aspsmembers.org/

Source: U.S. BUREAU OF LABOR STATISTICS

PSYCHIATRIC TECHNICIANS

OVERVIEW

Psychiatric technicians care for people who have mental or emotional conditions or developmental disabilities. Technicians typically monitor patients' conditions and provide therapeutic care, such as overseeing their medications.

Some psychiatric technicians provide care to patients who have severe developmental disabilities or mental health issues. Others work with patients undergoing rehabilitation for drug and alcohol addiction. Their work varies based on the types of patients they work with.

Psychiatric technicians work as part of a medical team under the direction of physicians or registered nurses. Other team members may include psychiatrists, psychologists, social workers, counselors, and therapists.

Psychiatric technicians typically do the following:

- Listen to patients' concerns, observe their behavior, and record their condition
- Report changes in patient health or behavior to medical staff
- Lead patients in therapeutic and recreational activities
- Provide medications and other treatments to patients, following instructions from doctors
- Help with patient intake and discharge
- Help patients with daily living activities
- Restrain patients who are or may become physically violent

Education Level

Postsecondary Non-Degree

Type of Area

Clinical

License or Certification

- Depends on State

Average Salary: $36k	Number of Jobs in 2021: 138,900
Average Hourly: $17/hr	Job Outlook in 2021: 9%
Salary Range: $26k to $56k	10y Change 2021 - 2031: 12,500

Education Requirements

- Education Program (1-2 years)

Work Environment

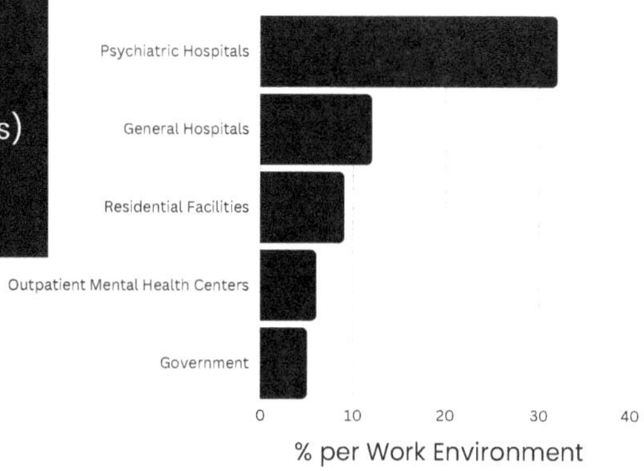

Note: Psychiatric aides help patients with mental or emotional conditions or developmental disabilities with their daily activities and ensure a safe and clean environment. Psychiatric aides typically need a high school diploma or equivalent.

Resources:

- American Association of Psychiatric Technicians: https://psychtechs.org/

Source: U.S. BUREAU OF LABOR STATISTICS

RADIATION THERAPISTS

OVERVIEW

Radiation therapists administer doses of radiation to patients who have cancer or other serious diseases.

Radiation therapists operate machines, such as linear accelerators, to deliver concentrated radiation therapy to the region of a patient's tumor. Radiation treatment may shrink or eliminate cancers and tumors.
Radiation therapists are part of the oncology teams that treat patients with cancer.

They often work with different specialists including Medical dosimetrists, Medical physicists, Oncology nurses, and Radiation oncologists.

Radiation therapists typically do the following:

- Explain treatment plans to the patient and answer questions about treatment
- Protect the patients and themselves from improper exposure to radiation
- Determine the location of tumors to ensure correct positioning of patients for administering each treatment
- Calibrate and operate the machine to treat the patient with radiation
- Monitor the patient to check for unusual reactions to the treatment

Education Level

Associate's Degree

Type of Area

Clinical

License or Certification

- State License

Average Salary: **$82k**
Average Hourly: **$39/hr**
Salary Range: **$61k to $128k**

Number of Jobs in 2021: **16,400**
Job Outlook in 2021: **6%**
10y Change 2021 - 2031: **1,000**

Education Requirements

- Associate's Degree (2 years) or Bachelor's Degree (4 years)

Work Environment

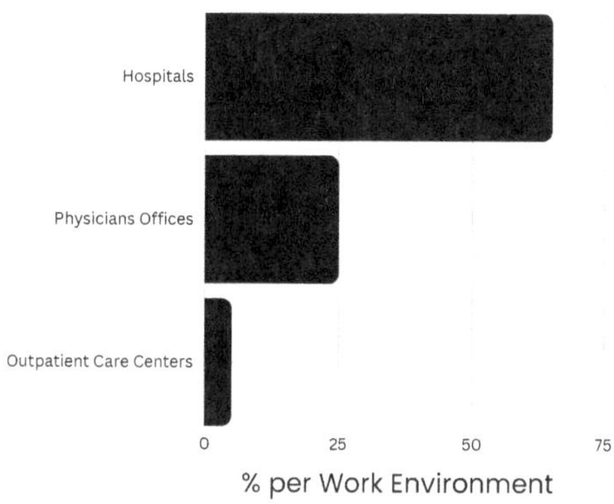

Resources:

- American Society of Radiologic Therapists: https://www.asrt.org/

Source: U.S. BUREAU OF LABOR STATISTICS

RADIOLOGIC TECHNOLOGISTS

OVERVIEW

Radiologic technologists, also known as radiographers, perform x-rays and other diagnostic imaging examinations on patients. Radiologic technologists are trained in the use of different types of medical diagnostic equipment.

They may choose to specialize, such as in x-ray, mammography, or computed tomography (CT) imaging. Some radiologic technologists provide a mixture for the patient to drink that allows soft tissue to be viewed on the images that the radiologist reviews.

Radiologic Technologists typically do the following:

- Adjust and maintain imaging equipment
- Follow precise orders from physicians on what areas of the body to image
- Prepare patients for procedures, including taking a medical history and shielding exposed areas that do not need to be imaged
- Position the patient and the equipment in order to get the correct image
- Operate the computerized equipment to take the images
- Work with physicians to evaluate the images and to determine whether additional images need to be taken

Education Level

Associate's Degree

Type of Area

Clinical

License or Certification

- Depends on State

Average Salary: **$77k**	**Number of Jobs in 2021:** **264,000**
Average Hourly: **$37/hr**	**Job Outlook in 2021:** **6%**
Salary Range: **$59k to $100k**	**10y Change 2021 - 2031:** **17,000**

Education Requirements

- Associate's Degree (2 years)

Work Environment

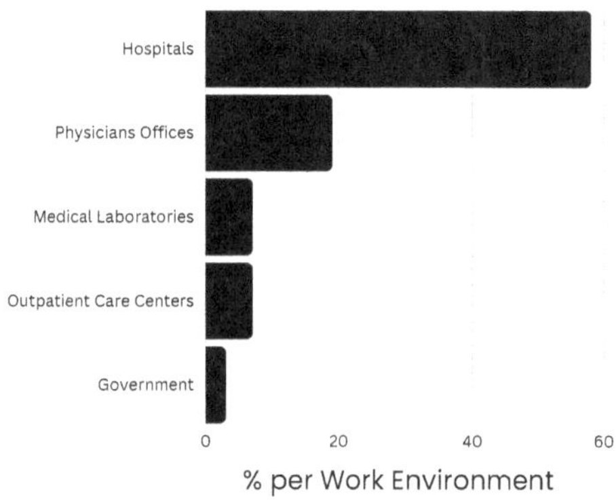

Resources:

- American Society of Radiologic Technologists: https://www.arrt.org/

Source: U.S. BUREAU OF LABOR STATISTICS

REGISTERED NURSES

OVERVIEW

Registered nurses (RNs) provide and coordinate patient care and educate patients and the public about various health conditions.

Most registered nurses work as part of a team with physicians and other healthcare specialists. Some registered nurses oversee licensed practical nurses, nursing assistants, and home health aides. Registered nurses' duties and titles often depend on where they work and the patients they work with.

Registered Nurses typically do the following:

- Assess patients' conditions
- Record patients' medical histories and symptoms
- Observe patients and record the observations
- Administer patients' medicines and treatments
- Set up plans for patients' care or contribute information to existing plans
- Consult and collaborate with doctors and other healthcare professionals
- Help perform diagnostic tests and analyze the results
- Teach patients and their families how to manage illnesses or injuries
- Explain what to do at home after treatment

Education Level

Bachelor's Degree

Type of Area

Clinical

License or Certification

- State License
- National Council Licensure Examination (NCLEX-RN)

Average Salary: $77k	Number of Jobs in 2021: 3,130,600
Average Hourly: $37/hr	**Job Outlook in 2021:** 6%
Salary Range: $59k to $120k	**10y Change 2021 - 2031:** 195,400

Education Requirements

- Associate's Degree (2 years) or
- Bachelor's Degree (4 years) or
- Education Program

Work Environment

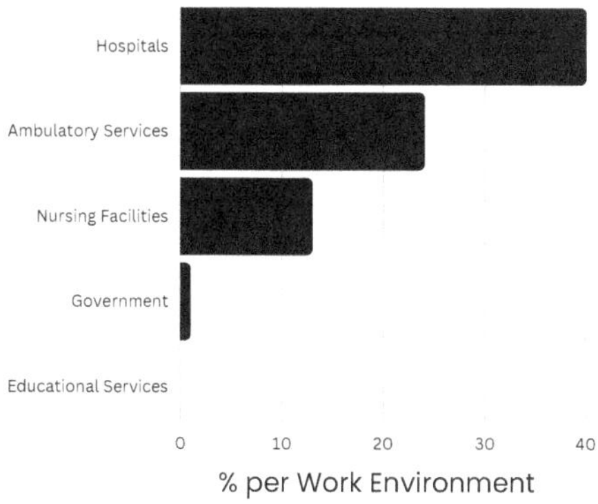

Note: Types of nurses include Addiction nurses, Cardiovascular nurses, Critical care nurses, Genetics nurses, Neonatal nurses, Nephrology nurses, Public health nurses, and Rehabilitation nurses. Some nurses do not work directly with patients, but they must still have an active registered nurse license. For example, they may work as nurse educators, healthcare consultants, or hospital administrators. Clinical nurse specialists (CNSs) are a type of advanced practice registered nurse (APRN).

Resources:

- American Nurses Association: https://www.nursingworld.org/

Source: U.S. BUREAU OF LABOR STATISTICS

REHABILITATION COUNSELORS

OVERVIEW

Rehabilitation counselors help people with physical, mental, developmental, or emotional disabilities live independently. They work with clients to overcome or manage the personal, social, or psychological effects of disabilities on employment or independent living.

Rehabilitation counselors help people with disabilities at various stages in their lives. Some work with students, to develop strategies to live with their disability and transition from school to work. Others help veterans cope with the mental or physical effects of their military service. Still others help elderly people adapt to disabilities developed later in life from illness or injury.

Rehabilitation Counselors typically do the following:

- Provide counseling to help clients adjust to their disability
- Evaluate clients' abilities, interests, experiences, skills, health, and education
- Develop a treatment plan for clients in consultation with other professionals
- Arrange for clients to obtain services
- Help employers understand the needs and abilities of people with disabilities, as well as laws and resources that affect people with disabilities
- Help clients develop their strengths and adjust to their limitations
- Locate resources that help clients live and work more independently
- Advocate for the rights of people with disabilities

Education Level

Master's Degree

Type of Area

Clinical

License or Certification

- Depends on Employment

Average Salary: $38k	Number of Jobs in 2021: 93,200
Average Hourly: $18/hr	Job Outlook in 2021: 11%
Salary Range: $28k to $65k	10y Change 2021 - 2031: 9,800

Education Requirements

- Bachelor's Degree (4 years)
- Master's Degree (2 years)

Work Environment

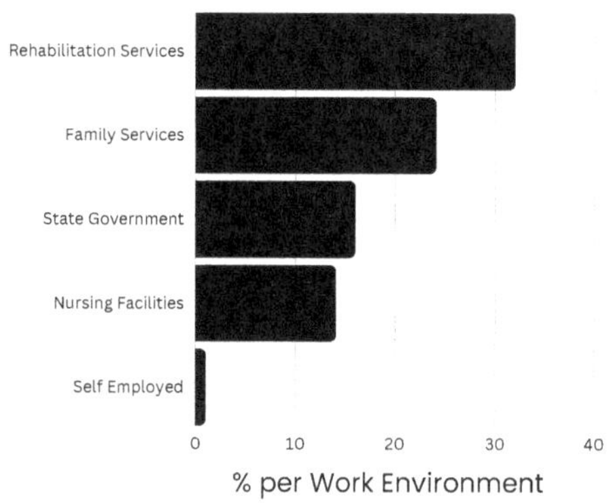

Resources:

- National Rehabilitation Counseling Association: https://nationalrehabcounselingassciation.wildapricot.org/
- American Rehabilitation Counseling Association: /https://www.arcaweb.org/

Source: U.S. BUREAU OF LABOR STATISTICS

RESPIRATORY THERAPISTS

OVERVIEW

Respiratory therapists care for patients who have trouble breathing. Their patients range from premature infants with undeveloped lungs to older adults whose lungs are diseased.

Respiratory therapists work closely with registered nurses, physicians and surgeons, and medical assistants. They use various tests to evaluate patients including pulmonary function tests. Respiratory therapists also perform treatment to clear airways for improved breathing.

Respiratory therapists in emergency settings may connect patients who cannot breathe on their own to ventilators that deliver oxygen to the lungs. They set up and monitor the equipment to ensure that the patient is receiving the correct amount of oxygen at the correct rate.

Respiratory therapists typically do the following:

- Interview and examine patients with breathing or cardiopulmonary disorders
- Consult with physicians about patients' conditions and developing treatment plans
- Perform diagnostic tests
- Treat patients using a variety of methods
- Monitor and record patients' progress
- Teach patients how to take medications and use equipment

Education Level

Associate's Degree

Type of Area

Clinical

License or Certification

- Depends on State

Average Salary: $61k	Number of Jobs in 2021: 135,800
Average Hourly: $29/hr	Job Outlook in 2021: 14%
Salary Range: $47k to $95k	10y Change 2021 - 2031: 18,400

Education Requirements

- Associate's Degree (2 years)

Work Environment

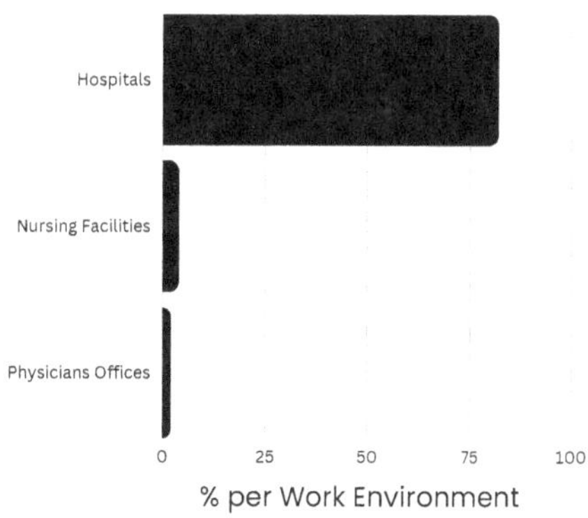

Resources:

- American Association of Respiratory Care: https://www.aarc.org/

Source: U.S. BUREAU OF LABOR STATISTICS

SOCIAL WORKERS

OVERVIEW

Social workers help individuals, groups, and families prevent and cope with problems in their everyday lives. Clinical social workers diagnose and treat mental, behavioral, and emotional problems.

They help with a wide range of situations, such as adopting a child, being diagnosed with a terminal illness, or preventing and treating substance abuse. Some social workers get involved at a broad level to help community organizations and policymakers develop or improve social programs, services, and conditions. Social workers advocate or raise awareness with and on behalf of their clients and constituents.

Social workers who are licensed to diagnose and treat mental, behavioral, and emotional disorders are called clinical social workers (CSW), licensed clinical social workers (LCSW), or have a similar title.

Social workers typically do the following:

- Identify people and communities in need of help
- Assess clients' needs, situations, strengths, and support networks to determine their goals
- Help clients adjust to changes and challenges in their lives, such as illness, divorce, or unemployment
- Research, refer, and advocate for community resources to assist and improve a client's well-being
- Respond to crisis situations such as child abuse and mental health emergencies
- Monitor clients' situations, and follow up to ensure that they have improved
- Provide psychotherapy services

Education Level

Bachelor's Degree

Type of Area

Clinical and Non-Clinical

License or Certification

- State License

Average Salary: **$50k**
Average Hourly: **$24/hr**
Salary Range: **$36k to $82k**

Number of Jobs in 2021: **708,100**
Job Outlook in 2021: **9%**
10y Change 2021 - 2031: **64,000**

Education Requirements

- Bachelor's Degree (4 years)
- Master's Degree (2 years), optional

Work Environment

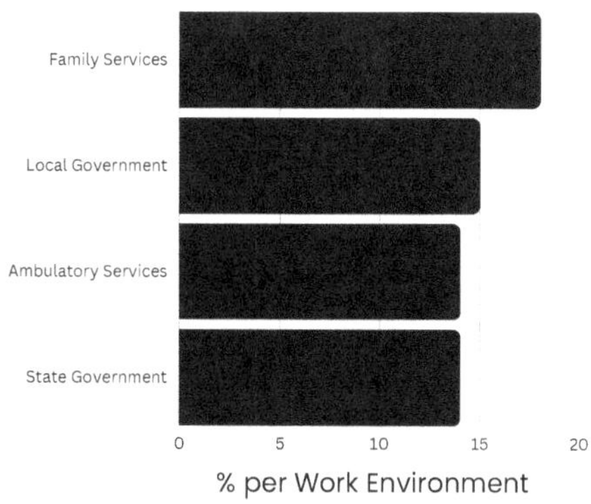

Note: Examples of types of social workers include Child and family social workers, School social workers, Healthcare social workers, and Mental health and substance abuse social workers.

Resources:

- National Association of Social Workers: https://www.socialworkers.org/
- Clinical Social Worker Association: http://www.clinicalsocialworkassociation.org/

Source: U.S. BUREAU OF LABOR STATISTICS

SPEECH LANGUAGE PATHOLOGISTS

OVERVIEW

Speech-language pathologists (sometimes called speech therapists) assess and treat people who have speech, language, voice, and fluency disorders. They also treat clients who have problems swallowing.

Speech-language pathologists work with clients who have speech and language problems, including related cognitive or social communication problems. Clients may have difficulty speaking, have problems with rhythm and fluency, such as stuttering, or have problems understanding language. Speech-language pathologists may select alternative communication systems and instruct clients in their use.

Speech-language pathologists typically do the following:

- Evaluate levels of speech, language, or swallowing difficulty
- Create and carry out an individualized treatment plan that addresses specific functional needs
- Teach clients how to make sounds, improve their voices, and maintain fluency
- Help clients improve vocabulary and sentence structure
- Work with clients to develop and strengthen the muscles used to swallow
- Counsel clients and their families on how to cope with communication and swallowing disorders

Education Level

Master's Degree

Type of Area

Clinical

License or Certification

- State License

Average Salary: **$79k**	**Number of Jobs in 2021:** **159,800**
Average Hourly: **$38/hr**	**Job Outlook in 2021:** **21%**
Salary Range: **$51k to $125k**	**10y Change 2021 - 2031:** **34,000**

Education Requirements

- Bachelor's Degree (4 years)
- Master's Degree (2 years)

Work Environment

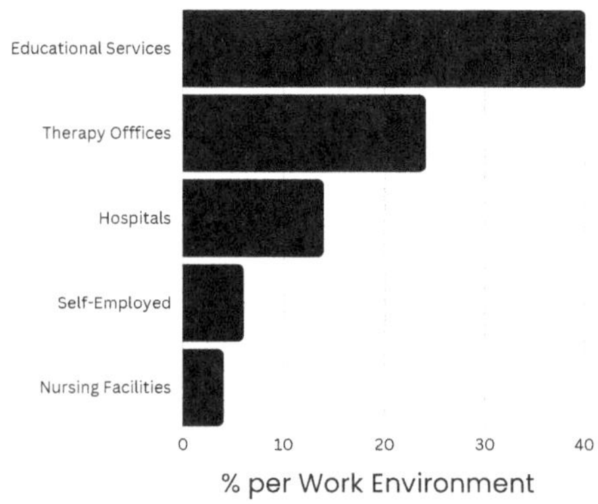

Resources:

- American Speech-Language-Hearing Association: https://www.asha.org/

Source: U.S. BUREAU OF LABOR STATISTICS

SURGICAL TECHNOLOGISTS

OVERVIEW

Surgical technologists help with surgical operations. Surgical technologists, also called operating room technicians, prepare operating rooms, arrange equipment, and help doctors and first assistants during surgeries.

Before an operation, surgical technologists prepare the operating room by setting up surgical instruments, equipment, solutions, and medications. Surgical technologists also bring patients to the operating room and get them ready for surgery by positioning them on the table, covering them with sterile drapes, and washing and disinfecting incision sites.

During an operation, surgical technologists pass the sterile instruments and supplies to surgeons and first assistants. They might hold retractors, hold internal organs in place during the procedure, or set up robotic surgical equipment. After the operation is complete, surgical technologists may apply bandages and other dressings to the incision site.

Surgical technologists typically do the following:

- Prepare operating rooms for surgery
- Sterilize equipment and make sure that there are adequate supplies for surgery
- Ready patients for surgery, such as by washing and disinfecting incision sites
- Help surgeons during surgery by passing them instruments and other sterile supplies
- Count supplies to ensure that no foreign objects are retained in patients
- Maintain a sterile environment to prevent patient infection

Education Level

Post Secondary Non-Degree

Type of Area

Clinical

License or Certification

- Depends on Employment

Average Salary: **$48k**	**Number of Jobs in 2021:** **110,700**
Average Hourly: **$23/hr**	**Job Outlook in 2021:** **6%**
Salary Range: **$36k to $75k**	**10y Change 2021 - 2031:** **6,500**

Work Environment

Education Requirements

- Associate's Degree (2 years)

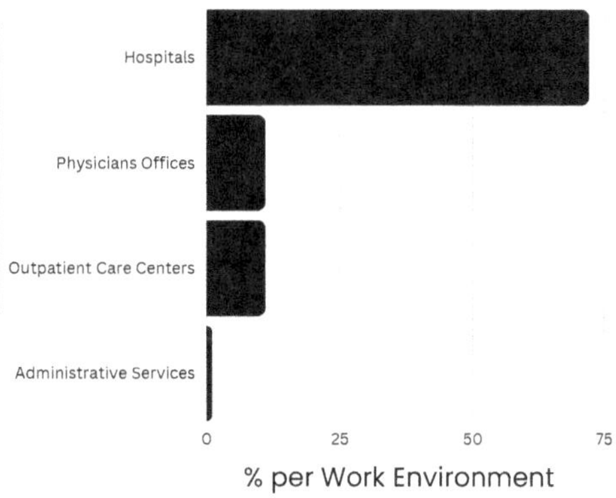

Note: Surgical assistants, also called surgical first assistants, help surgeons with tasks such as making incisions, placing clamps, and closing surgical sites. Surgical assistants have a hands-on role, directly assisting surgeons during a procedure. For example, they may help to suction the incision site or suture a wound.

Resources:

- Association of Surgical Technologists: https://www.ast.org/

Source: U.S. BUREAU OF LABOR STATISTICS

VETERINARIANS

OVERVIEW

Veterinarians care for the health of animals and work to protect public health. They diagnose, treat, and research medical conditions and diseases of pets, livestock, and other animals.

Veterinarians treat the injuries and illnesses of pets and other animals with a variety of medical equipment, including surgical tools and x-ray and ultrasound machines. They provide treatment for animals that is similar to the services a physician provides to humans.

Veterinarians typically do the following:

- Examine animals to assess their health and diagnose problems
- Treat and dress wounds
- Perform surgery on animals
- Test for and vaccinate against diseases
- Operate medical equipment, such as x-ray machines
- Advise animal owners about general care, medical conditions, and treatments
- Prescribe medication
- Euthanize animals

Education Level

Doctorate Degree

Type of Area

Clinical

License or Certification

- State License
- North American Veterinary Licensing Exam

Average Salary: $100k	Number of Jobs in 2021: 86,300
Average Hourly: $48/hr	Job Outlook in 2021: 19%
Salary Range: $60k to $165k	10y Change 2021 - 2031: 16,800

Education Requirements

- Bachelor's Degree (4 years)
- Doctor of Veterinary Medicine (4 years, DVM)

Work Environment

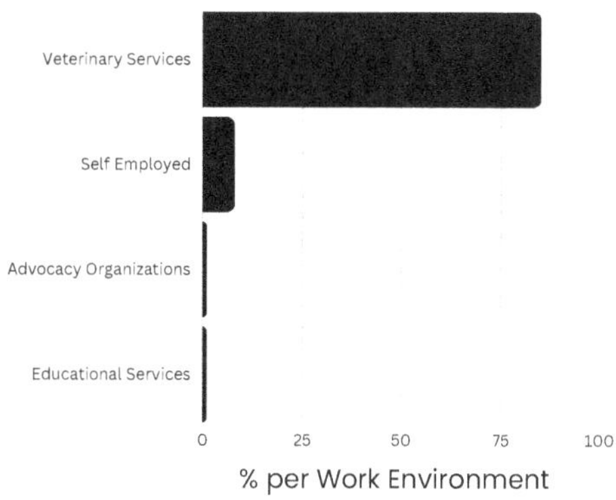

Note: Examples of types of veterinarians include Companion animal veterinarians, Food animal veterinarians, and Food safety and inspection veterinarians.

Resources:

- American Veterinary Medical Association: https://www.avma.org/

Source: U.S. BUREAU OF LABOR STATISTICS

VETERINARY ASSISTANTS AND LABORATORY ANIMAL CARETAKERS

OVERVIEW

Veterinary assistants and laboratory animal caretakers handle routine animal care and help scientists, veterinarians, and others with their daily tasks.

Veterinary assistants and laboratory animal caretakers also provide nursing care before surgery and other medical procedures. They may prepare equipment and pass surgical instruments and materials to veterinarians during surgery. They also move animals during testing and other procedures.

Veterinary assistants typically help veterinarians and veterinary technologists and technicians treat injuries and illnesses of animals.

Laboratory animal caretakers' daily tasks include feeding animals, cleaning kennels, and monitoring animals.

Veterinary assistants and Laboratory animal caretakers typically do the following:

- Feed, bathe, and exercise animals
- Clean and disinfect cages, kennels, and examination and operating rooms
- Restrain animals during examination and laboratory procedures
- Monitor and care for animals after surgery
- Help provide emergency first aid to sick and injured animals
- Give medication or immunizations that veterinarians prescribe
- Assist in collecting blood, urine, and tissue samples

Education Level

High School Diploma

Type of Area

Clinical

License or Certification

- None

Average Salary: $29k	Number of Jobs in 2021: 103,500
Average Hourly: $14/hr	Job Outlook in 2021: 19%
Salary Range: $22k to $38k	10y Change 2021 - 2031: 20,000

Education Requirements

- On the Job Training

Work Environment

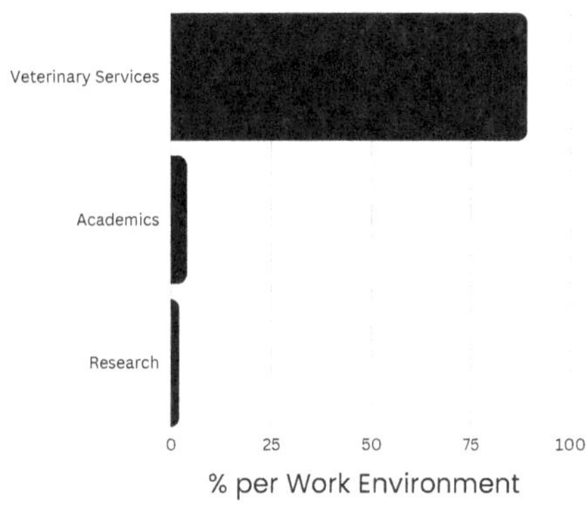

Resources:

- American Veterinary Medical Association: https://www.avma.org/

Source: U.S. BUREAU OF LABOR STATISTICS

VETERINARY TECHNOLOGISTS AND TECHNICIANS

OVERVIEW

Veterinary technologists and technicians do medical tests that help diagnose animals' injuries and illnesses. In addition to helping veterinarians during animal exams, veterinary technologists and technicians do a variety of clinical, care, and laboratory tasks. Veterinary technologists and technicians who work in research-related jobs ensure that animals are handled carefully and are treated humanely.

Veterinary technologists typically work in more advanced research-related jobs and work primarily in a laboratory setting. Veterinary technicians generally work in private clinical practices under the guidance of a licensed veterinarian. Although they do some of their work in a laboratory, technicians also talk with animal owners.

Veterinary technologists and technicians typically do the following:

- Observe the behavior and condition of animals
- Provide nursing care or emergency first aid to animals
- Bathe animals, clip nails or claws, and brush or cut animals' hair
- Restrain animals during exams or procedures
- Administer anesthesia to animals and monitor their responses
- Take x-rays and collect and perform laboratory tests
- Prepare animals and instruments for surgery
- Administer medications, vaccines, and treatments prescribed by a veterinarian

Education Level

Associate's Degree

Type of Area

Clinical

License or Certification

- State License
- Veterinary Technician National Examination (VTN

Average Salary: $36k	Number of Jobs in 2021: 122,800
Average Hourly: $17/hr	Job Outlook in 2021: 20%
Salary Range: $28k to $48k	10y Change 2021 - 2031: 24,100

Education Requirements

- Associate's Degree (2 years)
- Bachelor's Degree (4 years), optional

Work Environment

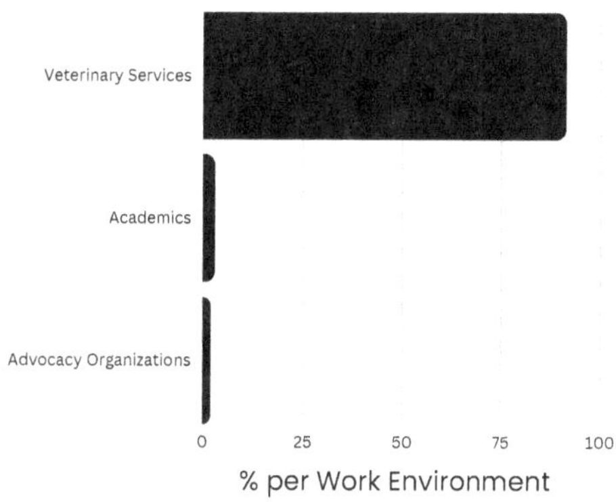

Note: Veterinary technologists and technicians may specialize in a particular discipline, such as dentistry, anesthesia, emergency and critical care, and zoological medicine.

Resources:

- American Veterinary Medical Association: https://www.avma.org/

Source: U.S. BUREAU OF LABOR STATISTICS

WHOLESALE AND MANUFACTURING SALES REPRESENTATIVES

OVERVIEW

Wholesale and manufacturing sales representatives sell goods for wholesalers or manufacturers to businesses, government agencies, and other organizations. They contact customers, explain the features of the products they are selling, negotiate prices, and answer any questions that their customers may have about the products.

Some wholesale and manufacturing sales representatives work with nonscientific products, such as food, office supplies, and clothing. Other representatives specialize in technical and scientific products, ranging from agricultural and mechanical equipment to computer and pharmaceutical goods.

Unlike retail sales workers, who sell goods directly to consumers, wholesale and manufacturing sales representatives deal with businesses, government agencies, and other organizations.

Wholesale and Manufacturing sales representatives typically do the following:

- Identify prospective customers
- Contact new and existing customers to discuss their needs and explain how specific products and services can meet these needs
- Help customers select products to meet customers' needs, product specifications, and regulations
- Emphasize product features that will meet customers' needs, and exhibit the capabilities and limitations of their products
- Answer customers' questions
- Negotiate prices and terms of sales and service agreements

Education Level

High School Diploma

Type of Area

Clinical

License or Certification

- Depends on State

Average Salary: **$62k**	**Number of Jobs in 2021:** **1,597,600**
Average Hourly: **$30/hr**	**Job Outlook in 2021:** **4%**
Salary Range: **$30k to $125k**	**10y Change 2021 - 2031:** **63,300**

Work Environment

Education Requirements

- On the Job Training
- Bachelor's Degree (4 years), optional
- Education Program, optional

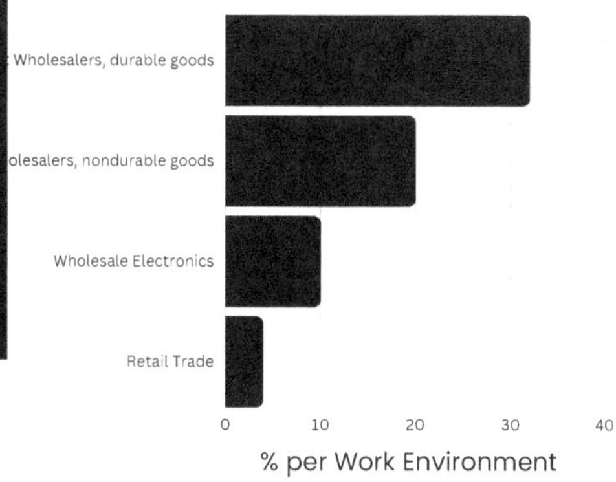

Note: Examples of types of wholesale and manufacturing sales representatives include Inside sales representatives and Outside sales representatives.

Source: U.S. BUREAU OF LABOR STATISTICS

www.ingramcontent.com/pod-product-compliance
Lightning Source LLC
LaVergne TN
LVHW022053200926
848481LV00003B/897
9798988939009